International Social Work Practice

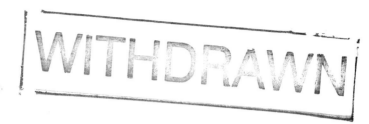
International Social Work Practice compares and contrasts divergent social work approaches in countries around the world, providing students with a unique perspective on social work as it is actually practised. Using case studies from frontline practitioners from across the globe, this innovative new textbook stimulates critical thinking about international social work practice issues.

Providing a review of both country-specific social work practices and universal social work issues, the text looks at a variety of core social work topics, framed here in terms of CSWE competencies. Set within a theoretical framework presented in the introductory chapter, the subjects covered include:

- child welfare
- intimate partner violence
- family conflict and communication
- elder care
- substance abuse
- trauma.

Each chapter presents several case studies exploring a range of issues within the broader topic. Each case study is commented on by two narratives from social work academics and practitioners from different countries, providing different cultural perspectives. Additional case studies are available online, via http://www.routledge.com/books/details/9780415783668/

Taking a practical hands-on approach, this text includes a dedicated section for classroom use, with discussion questions, classroom exercises, and additional cases for your own analysis. It will be particularly useful to BSW and MSW students taking courses in international social work, practice, social welfare, and human behavior.

Joanna E. Bettmann is an Associate Professor and the MSW Program Director at the University of Utah College of Social Work, USA.

Gloria Jacques is an Associate Professor in the Department of Social Work at the University

Caren J. Fro Social Work Research and a
Research Prof lege of Social Work, USA.

International Social Work Practice

Case Studies from a Global Context

Edited by Joanna E. Bettmann, Gloria Jacques, and Caren J. Frost

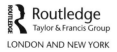

Routledge
Taylor & Francis Group

LONDON AND NEW YORK

First published 2013
by Routledge
2 Park Square, Milton Park, Abingdon, Oxon OX14 4RN

Simultaneously published in the USA and Canada
by Routledge
711 Third Avenue, New York, NY 10017

Routledge is an imprint of the Taylor & Francis Group, an informa
business

British Library Cataloguing in Publication Data
A catalogue record for this book is available from the British Library

Library of Congress Cataloging in Publication Data
International social work practice : case studies from a global context / edited
by Joanna E. Bettmann, Gloria Jacques, and Caren J. Frost. -- 1st ed.
p. cm.
1. Social service--Vocational guidance. I. Bettmann, Joanna E. II. Jacques,
Gloria. III. Frost, Caren J.
HV10.5.148 2013
361.3'2--dc23
2012024455

ISBN: 978-0-415-78365-1 (hbk)
ISBN: 978-0-415-78366-8 (pbk)
ISBN: 978-0-203-07650-7 (ebk)

Typeset in Goudy
by Fakenham Prepress Solutions, Fakenham, Norfolk NR21 8NN

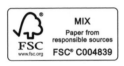

Printed and bound by CPI Group (UK) Ltd, Croydon, CR0 4YY

Contents

Acknowledgements

Writing this book has been a wonderful, and most rewarding, learning experience. We have gained professionally as we have engaged with the collaborators on the case studies and analyses—and for that we sincerely thank our colleagues. We extend our gratitude especially to Isaac Karikari, Gabriela Saile Hernandez de Alba, Linda Mendenhall, Kimber Parry, and Rita Ntshutelang for their efforts on our behalf! We especially want to thank Delva Hommes for her support of our work and grounded feedback on our ideas. Their writing, editing, critical reflection, and endless hours transcribing the material have enabled us to successfully complete this book.

Biographic Information of Authors

Lisa Salma Abubakar (Ghana) BA is a social development officer at the Department of Social Welfare, Ashanti region of Ghana. She has eight years' experience in social work practice on issues of justice administration, child care and protection as well as community development.

Wilson Alexander Alvarado (El Salvador) MA is the director of Equipo Nahual, one of the few NGOs dedicated to community outreach with high risk youth and youth actively involved in gangs in El Salvador and Guatemala. He has an MA in Sports Psychology from Universidad Nacional de El Salvador. He has worked in outreach with local gang-involved youth for more than 10 years using harm reduction and human rights perspectives.

Troy Christian Andersen (USA) MSW, MS, LCSW, PhD candidate, is a dementia specialist social worker at the Center for Alzheimer's Care, Imaging and Research at the University of Utah and is also an instructor at the University of Utah College of Social Work. Mr Andersen has over 20 years of clinical social work practice. His current clinical and research focus is on proactive planning for care-related needs of individuals with progressive neurologic diseases.

Naina Athale (India) is pursuing her PhD and is an Assistant Professor in the School of Social Work at the Tata Institute of Social Sciences, Mumbai, India. She has over 25 years' experience as a social worker in the field of child protection and counseling.

Mika Barber (USA) is working on her MSW at the University of Utah College of Social Work, Salt Lake City, Utah.

Mark Edward Barr (USA) received his MSW from the University of Utah College of Social Work in Salt Lake City, Utah.

Nehami Baum (Israel) PhD is a Professor at the Louis and Gabi Weisfeld School of Social Work at Bar Ilan University in Israel.

Joanna E. Bettmann (USA) PhD is an Associate Professor and the MSW Program Director at the University of Utah College of Social Work. She conducts research in the area of attachment, wilderness therapy, and psychotherapy, and has presented her research nationally and internationally. She maintains a clinical social work practice working with adolescents and young adults in Salt Lake City, Utah.

Lynne Briggs (New Zealand and Australia) PhD is a registered social worker who recently accepted a position as Associate Professor of Social Work at Griffith University, Queensland, Australia. Lynne previously held a joint academic/clinical position with the University of Otago in New Zealand. She has over 20 years' clinical practice experience in mental health services. Her research interests are in the area of mental health with a focus on refugee and migrant resettlement.

Dimitrinka Bumbovska (Bulgaria) is Head of the Child Protection Department in Sofia. She is a qualified case manager and practice teacher at Sofia University. She has 20 years' experience as a practitioner and manager in the field of social work with children and families, and has numerous publications on Bulgarian practice in this area.

Rob Butters (USA) PhD, LCSW, is the Director of the Utah Criminal Justice Center and Assistant Professor of Social Work at the University of Utah. He researches crime, delinquency, restorative justice and sexual abuse. Dr Butters is a licensed clinician and has 20 years' experience in working with at-risk adolescents in institutional and outpatient settings.

Kwon Ho Choi (South Korea) is a PhD candidate at Yonsei University, School of Social Welfare, South Korea. He was a pediatric social worker at Severance Hospital. His research interests include social inclusion of childhood cancer survivors, adolescent suicide, substance abuse and family violence.

Narcedalia Pratt Cornejo (Mexico) SSW, MSW, is a medical social worker who has been working primarily with the elderly for over six years. She has also worked with minority adolescents.

József Csürke (Hungary) MA in Social Policy and PhD in Psychology, is an Assistant Professor of Social Work, Chair of the Department of Social Work and Social Policy at the University of Pecs. He is a licensed supervisor in social work. He has 15 years' experience in lecturing, and considerable work experience in clinical social work with clients in crisis situations and mental health counseling. He conducts research on existentialist aspects of psychosocial crisis.

Robin L. Davis (USA) PhD, LCSW, is an Assistant Professor/Lecturer of Social Work at the University of Utah, Salt Lake City, Utah. She has worked for 18 years with at-risk youth and with the juvenile justice system. Her primary area of research interest is with Pacific Islander communities.

Peter Dwumah (Ghana) MPhil is a Lecturer of Sociology and Social Work at Kwame Nkrumah University of Science and Technology, Kumasi. He has seven years' experience in academia and currently conducts research on issues affecting youth, children and vulnerable groups in society. His research interests also include work and organizations.

Márta Erdős (Hungary) MA in Mental Health Counseling and PhD in Social Communication is an Associate Professor in Social Work and Head of Social Innovation and Evaluation Center at the University of Pecs. She worked at a Crisis and Counseling Centre for five years and in an addiction treatment center for five years. Her area of research is generativity in the context of the post-communist state.

Caren J. Frost (USA) PhD, MPH, is the Director of International Social Work Research and a Research Professor at the University of Utah College of Social Work. Her research areas are on ethnography, social-cultural aspects of breast cancer, and women's reproductive health.

Katy Gandevia (India) PhD is a Professor and Programme Convenor in the School of Social Work at the Tata Institute of Social Sciences (TISS) in Mumbai, where she coordinates medical and counseling services. She is on various national and international boards, has presented papers at various forums, and has published articles and books.

Ruth Gerritsen-McKane (USA) PhD, LCSW, is an Associate Professor/Lecturer of Social Work at the University of Utah. She is committed to the empowerment of vulnerable populations through education, and currently is part of a team researching the potential of global distance education.

Chanar Goodrich (Mongolia) MSW, has five years' experience working with Juvenile Justice Services for the State of Utah. In addition, she is the project coordinator for the University of Utah's study abroad projects in Mongolia.

Juha Hämäläinen (Finland) has a PhD in Social Policy, is a Professor of Social Work, especially Social Pedagogy, and Head of the Department of Social Sciences at the University of Eastern Finland. His research and teaching interests are in the theory and history of ideas of social work, ethics of social work, comparative social work, child welfare, youth research, and parenthood research.

Darsell M. Harris (USA) is the clinical manager in the Bureau of Juvenile Justice Services, Pennsylvania Department of Public Welfare.

Gabrielle Hesk (UK) Dip SW, PGCE, is a Lecturer in Social Work at the University of Salford. She is a qualified social worker with over 21 years' experience in working with children and their families, residential child care, adoption and fostering and disability. She is currently researching the intersection of gender and race from a feminist perspective and has a keen interest in women and children as survivors of domestic abuse/violence and rape.

Jennifer Hughes (USA) PhD candidate, MSW, LISW-S, is the Department Chair and an Assistant Professor of Social Work at Bluffton University in Bluffton, Ohio. She has had a private social work counseling practice in Lima, Ohio for 17 years and currently is conducting research on unpaid caregiving with Multiple Sclerosis patients.

Jeanna Jacobsen (USA) LCSW is a PhD Candidate in the College of School Work at the University of Utah. She has worked as a crisis line clinician since 2004. Her dissertation research is on the intersection of sexuality and spirituality with focus on sexual minorities and religious identity development.

Gloria Jacques (Botswana) has a Masters degree in Social Science from the University of Cape Town. She has practiced social work in England, Zambia, and South Africa and lectured in the discipline at the universities of Cape Town and Botswana (where she now resides). Her research interests are child welfare (notably statutory foster care), management and supervision in the human services, and human rights with particular reference to sexual minority groups. She is an Associate Professor in the Department of Social Work at the University of Botswana.

Hena John-Fisk (India) MSW, PhD candidate in Social Work at the University of Utah, has nine years' experience working with children, adolescents and adults in schools, red-light areas, and community settings.

She has worked with women and children infected with HIV/AID. Currently, she is conducting research about needs and experiences of prostitutes and their children.

Anish K. R. (India) M Phil, PhD, is an Assistant Professor of Social Work at the Rajagiri College of Social Sciences, Kerala, India. He has 13 years' experience working with families and children in clinical social work settings, and offers consultancy services for the National AIDS Control Organization. His areas of research include life skills, mental health rehabilitation, and the effectiveness of direct practice methods.

Sharvari Karandikar (India) PhD began her career practicing as a counselor for sex workers and victims of sex trafficking in Mumbai, India. During her PhD program in social work at the University of Utah, and through her work at the Tata Institute of Social Sciences (TISS) in Mumbai and later at Ohio State University, she has focused her research efforts on issues related to the female victims of sex trafficking, particularly on gender-based violence, health and mental health issues. Dr Karandikar's current research relates to egg donation and international surrogacy, as well as medical tourism and its impact on women.

Isaac Karikari (Ghana) received his MSW from the University of Utah, College of Social Work and is currently pursuing a PhD at Indiana University-Purdue University Indianapolis. He has a BA in Sociology and Social Work from the Kwame Nkrumah University of Science and Technology (KNUST) Kumasi.

Susan Kern (USA) received her MSW from the University of Utah College of Social Work in Salt Lake City, Utah.

Hyun Sook Kim (South Korea) PhD, RN, MSN, MSW, has been a Professor of Social Welfare at the Korea National University of Transportation (previously Chungju National University) since 2000. She has eight years' experience working in long-term care facilities, pediatrics wards and psychiatric units as a registered nurse in both America and Korea. Currently, she conducts research on end-of-life care and depression in the elderly.

Yong-Jung Kwon (South Korea) MSW, PhD, is an Executive Director of Konyang Buyeo Nursing Home. He has 15 years' experience working with the elderly in long term care facilities, and currently conducts research about program development and evaluation for care for the elderly.

Agnes Koon-chui Law (China) is a Professor at Sun Yat-sen University in China.

Natalie Lecy (USA) received her MSW from the University of Utah College of Social Work, Salt Lake City, Utah. Currently, she works as a clinical social worker in hospital and hospice settings.

Leena Leinonen (Finland) MA is a social work lecturer at the University of Eastern Finland.

Duane J. Luptak (USA) MSW, LCSW, is an Assistant Professor/Lecturer of Social Work at the University of Utah. He has over 20 years of experience working with adults with serious and persistent mental illness, and is currently a practicum coordinator at the College of Social Work.

Marilyn Luptak (USA) PhD, MSW, is a John A. Hartford Faculty Scholar in Geriatric Social Work and Assistant Professor of Social Work at the University of Utah. She brings 25 years of practice experience to her scholarly work to improve the health and well-being of older adults and their families.

Mandi MacDonald (Ireland) MSW, MRes is a Lecturer in Social Work at Queens University Belfast. She has 10 years' experience in statutory social work with children and families, and currently researches adoptive parenting and post-adoption contact.

József Madácsy (Hungary) MA in Philosophy, MSW, PhD student in Cultural Anthropology, is an Assistant Professor in Social Work at the University of Pecs. He has several years' experience working with learning/physical disabilities. His area of research interest is recovery from addictions.

Tumani Malinga-Musamba (Botswana) BSW, MSW, is a lecturer in the Department of Social Work, University of Botswana. She worked in a hospital setting before joining the university. Her research interests are HIV and AIDS, social work in health settings and life skills.

Nikoletta Mándi (Hungary) MA in Social Policy, is an Assistant in Social Work at the University of Pecs. She is a PhD candidate in Cultural Anthropology at the University of Pecs. She specializes in family care and family protection and is a qualified family therapist. She worked in a family help center for 10 years. Her area of research interest is addiction focusing on narrative identity changes during recovery.

Tobokane Manthai (Botswana) BSW, MSW, is working on her LCSW and pursuing a Master's degree in Science Operations Management focusing on industrial health and safety management. She is planning on completing a doctoral degree in social work to enhance her research agenda.

Kgosietsile Maripe (Botswana) BSW, MSW, is a lecturer in Social Work at the University of Botswana. He has 16 years' experience working in community social work settings and has taught courses on community development, disaster management, probation, and psychology for social workers. He is currently engaged in a PhD program on community resilience to disaster at the University of the North West, South Africa.

Margaret McKenzie (New Zealand) MA (Hons), Registered Social Worker, is a Senior Lecturer in the School of Social Services at Otago Polytechnic, in Dunedin. With more than 30 years' experience as a social work academic in New Zealand, she is a specialist in child and family mental health services. Her publications include explorations in family group conferencing, research with vulnerable groups, supervised contact, and community approaches to child protection.

Tirelo Modie (Botswana) BSW, MSW, and PhD, is a Senior Lecturer in the Department of Social Work at the University of Botswana.

Tshepo Mogapi (Botswana) BSW completed her studies at the University of Botswana.

Maithamako Molojwane (Kenya) has a Certificate in Social Work from the Kenya Institute of Administration and a Diploma in Social Policy and Administration from the University College of Swansea, University of Wales. She also has a BA in Psychology from the University College of Swansea, and an MA in Social Work from Columbia University. She is currently working as a counselor and is engaged in a PhD program in Counseling and Human Services at the University of Botswana.

Jamie Mortensen (USA) received her MSW from the University of Utah College of Social Work in Salt Lake City, Utah.

Georgina Mucsi (Hungary) MA in Social Work, is a PhD student in the Cultural Studies Doctoral programme at the University of Pecs. She is an Assistant Professor in Social Work and conducts research on hospice/palliative care. She has considerable work experience in community work with disadvantaged young people and she worked five years in hospice/palliative care.

Jillian Murphy (UK) MBA, BA, DASS, CQSW, is a Lecturer at Salford University. She has 35 years' experience in managing children and families in social work settings. She currently teaches in the Masters' degree program at Salford University, specializing in research skills and working with children and young people. She conducts research on disability and educational achievement.

Augustina Naami (Ghana) PhD is an Assistant Professor of Social Work at the University of Northern Iowa. Her research centers on disability, gender, and poverty. She has seven years' experience working with persons with disabilities, empowering them to advocate for their human rights and their socioeconomic and political development.

Yomei Nakatani (Japan) PhD, MSW, is an Associate Professor of Social Work at Japan Women's University, Kawasaki. He has worked as a hospital social worker and is engaged in research on gerontology topics such as caregiver issues.

Hannah Nam (South Korea) BS will graduate from the Pennsylvania State University College of Medicine in 2012 to pursue a residency in combined Internal Medicine/Pediatrics. She is fluent in both English and Korean. She is interested in the health care of minorities and the underserved, and is currently involved in research regarding health care of the geriatric population in a medical home setting.

Suryia Nayak (UK) CQWS, Ad Dip Counseling, is a Senior Lecturer in Social Work at the University of Salford. She is a feminist community activist, and is in the process of completing her PhD on Audre Lorde and the concept of difference.

Anita Neal (USA) received her MSW from the University of Utah College of Social Work in Salt Lake City, Utah.

Nthabiseng Nkwe (Botswana) has an academic background in social work and this has influenced her interest in various social issues such as human rights, HIV and AIDS and social development. She joined the Botswana Network on Ethics, Law and HIV/AIDS (BONELA) as an intern in 2004 and later became the project officer. Her work in the social policy field has involved extensive stakeholder collaboration in an effort to address the needs of divergent populations.

Nuelle Novik (Canada) MSW, PhD, RSW, is a Canadian social worker who currently works full time as an Assistant Professor with the Faculty of Social Work at the University of Regina, Saskatchewan, Canada. She also continues to practice as a social work therapist, working part-time as a counselor with a community-based agency.

Kwadwo Ofori-Dua (Ghana) is a Sociologist (MPhil Sociology) with a BA(Hons) in Sociology and Political Science. Currently, he serves as Lecturer at the Department of Sociology and Social Work, Kwame Nkrumah University of Science and Technology, Kumasi. He is also a PhD candidate in Social Work in the Department of Social Work,

University of Ghana, Legon researching the "The Effect of Weakening Social Support on the Aged."

Megan O'Keefe (USA) graduated from the University of Utah with an MA in Social Work. Her goal is to work as a substance abuse therapist.

René Olate (El Salvador) PhD is an Assistant Professor at the Ohio State University College of Social Work, USA. He has a BA degree in Social Work from Universidad de Concepción in Chile, and MA and PhD degrees in Social Work from Washington University. His research interests center on high risk youth, youth violence, Latino gangs and community and positive youth development.

Kwaku Osei-Hwedie (Botswana) PhD is Professor and Dean of the School of Governance and leadership at the Ghana Institute of Management and Public Administration (GIMPA), Achimota-Accra, Ghana. Formerly, he was Professor of Social Work at the University of Botswana.

So Rah Park (South Korea) PhD has been a psychiatric social worker at Severance Hospital since 1992. Her research interests include psycho-pathologies, especially schizophrenia, bipolar disorder, substance abuse, child abuse, domestic violence and the quality of life of patients with brain lesions and their families.

Pirjo Pölkki (Finland) PhD in Psychology, is Professor of Child Welfare at the Department of Social Sciences, University of Eastern Finland. She has taught psychology and child welfare for social work students for more than 20 years. Currently, she conducts research on processes and outcomes of child welfare, especially on outcomes of family support measures.

Henry Poduthase (India) MA, MSW, is currently a doctoral candidate at the University of Utah. With an MA in Economics and an MSW from Mahatma Gandhi University, he has worked for five years as Assistant Professor at Marian College Kuttikkanam, Kerala, India. Additionally, he has lectured on various topics in the BSW and MSW programmes at the University of Utah. His current research is focused on delinquent behavior and family systems.

Piia Puurunen (Finland) MA is a Junior Researcher at the University of Eastern Finland.

Morena J. Rankopo (Botswana) PhD is a Senior Lecturer at the University of Botswana, and former coordinator of the MSW program. He has 18 years' experience of teaching social work methods emphasizing culturally relevant social work education and practice.

Retnaningrum Retnaningtyas (Indonesia) SSosI is a social worker in the Office of Social Affairs in Indonesia. She received her undergraduate in Social Welfare at Islamic Community Development Program, Sunan Kalijaga Islamic University, Indonesia.

Andrea Ries (USA) CSW is a mental health therapist working with adults in the substance abuse field. She has worked in social work settings in Europe and the USA.

Christian Sarver (USA) is a Research Assistant at the College of Social Work, University of Utah, where she is pursuing a PhD. She has worked in victim services for 15 years.

Boitumelo Malebogo Segwabanyane (Botswana) BSW has 10 years' experience working with vulnerable groups such as People Living with HIV (PLWHIV), refugees, and asylum seekers. Currently, she is Acting Programs Manager for the Botswana Red Cross Society.

Mosarwa Segwabe (Botswana) BSW, MA, MPH, is presently employed in the orphaned and vulnerable children program, USAID PEPFAR.

Ritta Rossitsa Simonia (Bulgaria) PhD is an Assistant Professor at the Department of Social Work, Sofia University. She has 16 years' experience as a lecturer, trainer and consultant in Social Work Management and Educational Management courses and projects. Currently, she conducts research and publishes on Quality Management, Leadership, and Organizational Culture in social work organizations.

Refilwe Jeremiah Sinkamba (Botswana) MSW is a private consultant (Trainer) and a founder of Toro Community Youth Center. She has experience in working with adults and adolescents in a range of social work settings. She mentors youths on various issues including substance abuse and life development skills.

Carolyn Sterrett (USA) received her MSW from the University of Utah College of Social Work in Salt Lake City, Utah.

Lauren Stivers (USA) CSW has worked in Social Work for seven years. She previously worked in child protection and with homeless mentally ill and substance dependent clients. She currently works with children in an outpatient therapy unit.

Mari Suonio (Finland) MA is a Lecturer in social work at the University of Eastern Finland.

Eliot Sykes (USA) MSW is a Research Assistant at Utah Youth Village. He has nine years' experience working with adolescents and their families in various settings. Currently, he is developing clinically-based in-home interventions targeting depression, anxiety, eating disorder, and ADHD diagnoses.

Gábor Szöllősi (Hungary) has a MA in Law and Social Policy, as well as a PhD in Social Policy. He is an Associate Professor in Social Policy and is Program Leader of the Social Policy Masters' program at the University of Pecs. He significantly contributed to shaping the Hungarian system of social study programs and creating the Hungarian Child Protection Law.

Kayo Tobinaga (Japan) is a Clinical Psychologist who is currently lecturing at Kyushu Kyoritsu University, Fukuoka, Japan.

Derrik Tollefson (USA) PhD, MSW, is Associate Professor and Coordinator of the MSW program at Utah State University. He has conducted a number of studies on family violence and child welfare programs, has published in journals, contributed to book chapters, and presented at numerous national and international conferences. He teaches courses on family violence, child welfare, and social work practice.

Tara Tulley (USA) received her MSW from the University of Utah College of Social Work in Salt Lake City, Utah.

Roberta Uchoa (Brazil) PhD has been lecturing and developing qualitative and quantitative research in the arena of drug addiction and social policy for the last 10 years at the Federal University of Pernambuco, Brazil.

J. Matt Upton (USA) received his MSW from the University of Utah College of Social Work in Salt Lake City, Utah.

Riitta Väänänen (Finland) MA in Social Work, is the Director of Social and Health care Services at the Municipality of Keitele, Finland. She has worked for 16 years in the Department of Child Forensic Psychiatry in the University Hospital of Kuopio, and now leads the local Social and Health care Services, including Child Protection Social Work.

Marja Väänänen-Fomin (Finland) MA is a Lecturer in social work at the University of Eastern Finland.

Guido van de Luitgaarden (The Netherlands) PhD, BSW, is a Senior Lecturer/Researcher at Zuyd University in Maastricht, The Netherlands.

Margo van Rensburg (South Africa) has a nursing science degree majoring in community health. She spent a few years in Botswana where she was involved in community counseling. She currently assists in a medical practice in South Africa.

Riitta Vornanen (Finland) PhD is Professor of Social Work at the University of Eastern Finland, Department of Social Sciences. Her main interests in research are child welfare, social work with children and young people, and young people's experiences with security and risks. For the past 10 years, she has worked in teaching and developing a new kind of post-graduate education for social workers.

Cornelius Siswa Widyatmoko (Indonesia) MPsi is a Lecturer in the Psychology Department at Sanata Dharma University. He received his BA in Psychology and MA in Clinical Psychology from Gadjah Mada University. Besides teaching, he is involved in services for disaster survivors and youth, and also in research on sexuality.

1

Introduction – International Practice Issues

By Isaac Karikari and Joanna E. Bettmann

At the International Federation of Social Workers (IFSW) General Meeting in Montreal, Canada in 2000, the IFSW attempted to define social work. They asserted:

> The social work profession promotes social change, problem-solving in human relationships and the empowerment and liberation of people to enhance wellbeing. Utilizing theories of human behavior and social systems, social work intervenes at the points where people interact with their environments. Principles of human rights and social justice are fundamental to social work (IFSW, 2000).

This definition conveys the essential elements of social work in regard to its values, knowledge base, and modes of practice. However, some IFSW individuals and member associations expressed doubts regarding the accurate conveyance of the many variations and facets of social work (Hare, 2004). The above definition, however, significantly reflects the basic tenets of social work: the intrinsic worth of human beings which is the "central organizing and unifying concept of social work universally," and the attempt of social workers to intervene as humans interact with their environment (Hare, 2004, p. 409).

Scholars differ on what constitutes international social work, and offer various definitions for this term. Early definitions included the concepts of social work practice across nations, work with international organizations such as the International Labour Organization (ILO), and international conferences on social work (Healy & Thomas, 2007; Xu, 2006). Cross-cultural understanding, comparison, and application of international perspectives to local practice, as well as participation in policy and practice activities featured in these definitions too (Xu, 2006). Others assert that international social work refers to social work activities which are unlimited by national and cultural borders (Healy & Thomas, 2007). Still others state that international social work encompasses the policies and programs of international agencies doing social work (Healy & Thomas, 2007).

Many conclude that international social work generally includes practice that takes place in countries other than the home country of the social worker. Such practices include work with International Non-Governmental Organizations (INGOs) and international bodies such as the United Nations. This also includes the sharing and transfer of knowledge and ideas, especially from countries where social work is well established to those where it is less established (Hugman, Moosa-Mitha & Moyo, 2010; Xu, 2007).

The concept of international social work connotes work with populations or groups residing in a country other than their country of origin. Such groups include refugees and migrants (Hugman, Moosa-Mitha & Moyo, 2010). Another prominent feature of international social work practice is its consideration and analysis of how globalization affects human welfare (Hugman, Moosa-Mitha & Moyo, 2010). International social work may integrate global and local realities, out of which comes the term "glocal" (Hugman, Moosa-Mitha & Moyo, 2010, p. 631).

Our Book

Our book presents social work as practiced globally. Each chapter covers a different population common to social work practice: vulnerable children, abused women, substance-addicted adults, etc. Each chapter presents three fairly generic social work cases that might occur anywhere in the world. Then social work practitioners from two different countries present how they would each respond to the issues raised in the case study.

Therefore, the book details what social work practice in different international contexts looks like. The book illustrates how social work practice is both global and at the same time local, how social workers' interventions are both similar and different in varied country contexts. Such issues are important for all social work practitioners globally to consider. This book provides an international focus on social work with a concrete practice-based approach. The authors of the case studies and case analyses are practitioners in the social work field from countries in various regions throughout the world. These front-line practitioners have authored a contemporary book that compares and contrasts social work practices in Africa, Asia, the Middle East, Europe, Central America, South America, and the United States. It illustrates that although the purpose of social work is its practice, such practice is distinct in each country.

Before considering the specific topics presented in each chapter, we will review some of the roots and trends in worldwide social work practice.

Historical Development of Social Work

The exact time and place the social work profession began is difficult to ascertain (McPhail, 2004). Some trace the professional evolution of social work in the West to the second half of the nineteenth century when individuals, churches, and philanthropic and benevolent institutions engaged in activities aimed at bettering the conditions of the poor (Hugman, 1996; Kohs, 1966). Many believe the twentieth century marked the beginning and development of the profession. Social work first began as an activity by individuals who, in their own private capacities, offered aid and relief to the poor. Other groups and agencies engaged in these relief efforts, instituting interventions to help combat social problems such as poverty (Abrams & Curran, 2004; Dyeson, 2004; Healy, 2008; Jennissen & Lundy, 2005).

During the Victorian era in England, Samuel Barnett established the first settlement in 1884 at Toynbee Hall. The settlements were buildings where mostly poor and underprivileged people received assistance to alleviate the conditions of their poverty. The establishment of other settlements such as Women's University Settlement at Southwark, Oxford House in Bethnal Green, and Mansfield House in Canning Town, all in England, followed later (Herrick, 2005; Webb, 2007). These settlements served many purposes, such as being a means of promoting the social integration of the poor and the rich. Later on, social reformers like Jane Adams, Lillian Wald, and Robert Woods replicated the concept of settlement houses in the United States, working primarily with impoverished populations (Herrick, 2005).

In Canada too, settlement houses were a feature of the earliest development of social work. Some of the settlement houses in Canada were Women's University Settlement at McGill University, Montreal in 1891, and University Settlement at the University of Toronto in 1910. These houses were affiliated with universities, affording students opportunities to work with the poor as part of their education (Jennissen & Lundy, 2005). Religious beliefs and practices were fundamental to the development of social welfare services in ancient and early European societies such as Italy's Rome and Victorian-era England (Kohs, 1966). In very much the same way, the motivation for the establishment of some of these settlements in Europe was religious (Webb, 2007). Similarly, in Canada, Christian ideals inspired the provision of social services and the models of practice adopted in the settlement houses (Graham, 2005; Jennissen & Lundy, 2005).

These early developments represented humanitarian efforts that preceded the formal profession of social work. Before the development of the profession (of social work), societies took responsibility for the welfare needs of their members. In ancient Egypt, Babylon, and Rome, some texts, scripts, and precepts underscored the need for practices that ensured the well-being of the populace. They included references to segments of the population such as the widowed and the orphaned (Kohs, 1966). Such societies developed systems and structures for the provision of the primary needs of their people (Austin, 1983; Garvin & Tropman, 1998).

In England, the Poor Laws, the Poor Law Reform of 1834, and the Royal Commission of 1909 attempted to regulate welfare services. For example, the English Poor Law of 1601 made the government responsible for the welfare of the poor. Prior to this, religious authorities mainly took responsibility for the care of the poor (Garvin & Tropman, 1998). The Poor Law Reform of 1834 resulted in the stigmatization of the poor. This law brought an end to existing systems for providing relief under which the poor could receive aid without having to be in institutional or residential settings (Garvin & Tropman, 1998, p. 7). The 1834 reform resulted in the creation of workhouses, places where those lacking a means of support and livelihood received aid, and the categorization of the poor into the deserving poor and the undeserving poor. At this time, citizens were blamed for their poverty; being poor and receiving public assistance was considered an admission of one's failure. Further, being poor became synonymous with a low moral status and earned one a bad reputation (Garvin & Tropman, 1998).

In both England and the US, the emergence of the profession of social work is tied to the events and developments of this period. The efforts of the Charity Organization Society movement and an increase in the use of scientific methods by the settlement houses towards equipping people with skills were notable landmarks as they represented concerted efforts in dealing with social problems (Garvin & Tropman, 1998; Kohs, 1966).

Gender Roles within the Social Work Profession

In the early stages of the profession's development, women performed most social work activities (Austin, 1983). However, the popularly presented view of social work as a female-dominated profession, with its co-founders being Jane Addams and Mary Richmond, is inaccurate (McPhail, 2004). Such presentations fail to take into account the complexities surrounding the development of the profession. Women were prominent in the founding of the profession, but they did not do it alone (McPhail, 2004).

For instance, in Canada the combined efforts of both men and women were critical to the profession's development. The women mainly engaged in primary practice and the provision of services while the men played roles in policy development relevant to social work and social welfare (Jennissen & Lundy, 2005). In the history of Canadian social work, men often made their way into the social work field through other fields of study and academic disciplines such as economics and political science (Jennissen & Lundy, 2005). Such men generally secured positions in academic institutions, government agencies, and consultancies, and thus influenced practice through policy development (Jennissen & Lundy, 2005). These men often occupied managerial and leadership positions (McPhail, 2004).

Professionalization of Social Work

While social work practice has its roots in the nineteenth and twentieth centuries, its professionalization happened later. It is worth noting that social work's professional status has, at times, been the subject of contention (Weiss, Spiro, Sherer & Korin-Langer, 2004). The basis for this contention included factors such as the lack of a theoretical and knowledge base for practice and exclusivity in performing social services. Over time, this has changed as social work developed theoretical foundations for practice. Nevertheless, the level of professionalization varies from country to country (Weiss, Spiro, Sherer & Korin-Langer, 2004).

One prominent incident in social work's early beginnings was when American Abraham Flexner in 1915 raised questions about the professional status of social work. Flexner, a prominent person in US medical education, stated at the National Conference on Charities and Correction that social work did not fully meet all the requirements needed to be classified as a profession. He compared social work to established professions such as medicine, law, and painting. As the assistant secretary to the General Education Board, his opinions commanded influence (Austin, 1983).

Developing modules for training people as social workers played an important role in establishing social work as a profession. In the 1890s, US leaders such as Anna Dawes and Mary Richmond raised the idea of the establishment of schools for people whose work was offering aid to the poor. This idea led to the creation of social work schools in Chicago, New York, Boston, Philadelphia, and St. Louis at the beginning of the twentieth century (Stuart, 2005). In 1897, Mary Richmond, then the director of the Baltimore Charity Organization, called for an organized form of training (Austin, 1983). Subsequently, Edward Devine of the New York Charity Organization Society started a summer training program in 1898 for social work practitioners. Mary Richmond served as an instructor in Devine's training program. This training program was actually a precursor to year-long social work training programs (Austin, 1983). Under the auspices of foundations such as the Rockefeller philanthropies, the Russell Sage Foundation, and the Commonwealth Fund, the schools encouraged a scientific conceptualization of social problems (Stuart, 2005).

Another important landmark in the professionalization of US social work was the creation of the National Association of Social Workers (NASW). Formed in 1955 by a merger of seven US professional social work bodies, NASW formed another strong group which advocated for the professionalization and formal education of social workers. Despite these developments, research in social work education still remained a prominent issue because it was essential to establishing a strong knowledge base and keeping practitioners abreast of current trends. Doctorates in social work thus became increasingly popular in the US.

The first university social work class took place at New York's Columbia University in 1898. In 1919, the Association of Training Schools of Professional Social Work was founded (Dyeson, 2004). The American Association of Schools of Social Work (ASSW), founded in 1921, initially made professional education the minimum requirement for social workers and subsequently made graduate education the requirement. In the South and Midwest US, educators formed the National Association of Schools of Social Administration (NASSA) which promoted undergraduate education (Stuart, 2005). These two associations, the ASSW and NASSA, merged to become the Council on Social Work Education (CSWE) in 1952 (Stuart, 2005). CSWE aimed to set standards for the standardization and professionalization of social work education, a mission which it continues today.

The US Great Depression also had some effects on the social work profession's historical development. The Great Depression was a socio-economic crisis that had a debilitating effect on various sectors of the economy and social life, placing a great strain on the production of goods and services. Beginning in 1929, it lasted through the 1930s (Crafts & Fearon, 2010; Graham, Hazarika & Narasimhan, 2011). During the Great Depression, welfare activities that used to be provided by charities and philanthropic organizations became government-regulated services. The US government then began to enact policies and develop structures to streamline welfare services and activities. One example of this is the US Social Security Act of 1935 which, in addition to offering federal assistance, regulated state programs regarding the provision of social services (Stuart, 2005). Under the Social Security Act, the government established facilities to provide public assistance to the aged and the poor and needy (Wedemeyer & Moore, 1966).

Notably, social work existed in the 1920s in Eastern Europe (Lorenz, 2008). In Poland, for instance, Helena Radlinska founded a school of social work in 1925. Under later communist regimes, some social work practices were still in vogue. Social work even existed under its "Western" title in the former Yugoslavia (Lorenz, 2008, p.13). The use of this title was a political tactic, part of the government's efforts to seek an audience with the United Nations, as well as garnering support from US agencies for social work development (Lorenz, 2008).

The Influence of Colonialism and Politics on the Rise of Social Work

The introduction of social work to non-Western countries, notably in Africa and Asia, occurred through the efforts and activities of colonial powers in the twentieth century (Kreitzer & Wilson, 2010). Social work in Ghana has its roots in the British social welfare system introduced during the colonial period (Kreitzer & Wilson, 2010). Similarly, Vietnamese social work has colonial French and American influences (Oanh, 2002), as does Zimbabwean social work whose roots are in its colonial and apartheid periods (Molodovan & Moyo, 2007). In most of these countries, social work started during the colonial period as an initiative of colonial governments. As a result, it was often patterned after the form of social work practiced in the country of the colonialists (Hugman, 1996). The link between social work in Africa and colonialism may be responsible for the development of Eurocentric models in social work practice in African nations (Mwansa, 2011).

Notably, Western social work continues to influence social work in these regions. This occurs mostly because many social workers in Africa and Asia receive training in Western universities and institutions of higher education. It thus happens that they return to their home countries with Western-based education and ideals. This continues to happen despite the existing differences in addressing the social realities of these regions (Gray & Fook, 2004; Kreitzer & Wilson, 2010). Notably, the ethical codes and values employed in social work practice in most Western states often run counter to the values and ideals of various developing countries. With these differences, the direct transfer of knowledge and skills from Western nations for practice in developing nations will therefore be a misfit (Al-Krenawi, 1999; Lough, 2009). The individualist perspective of industrialized nations and the collectivist perspective of most developing nations also shape the problem solving models used in these societies. In collectivistic cultures, much value is placed on connectedness and interdependence among individuals compared to individualistic cultures where much emphasis is placed on asserting one's independence from others (Markus & Kitayama, 1991). Hence in developing nations like Ghana, the family (including extended family members) as a social unit plays a prominent role in ensuring the well-being of its members (Kreitzer & Wilson, 2010). Thus, the modification and adaptation of Western-based social work knowledge and skills is necessary to ensure that social work practices suit the local context of the places where they are being applied (Soliman & Elmegied, 2010). However, in countries like Botswana, the effect of HIV and AIDS has negatively impacted the family's traditional role of caring for its members and necessitated the development of more Western methods of coping, especially in the field of child care (Jacques, 2011).

Political developments at certain points in time affected the historical growth of social work. In Europe, communist regimes caused some institutions of learning to be closed down in places like Poland, while in Romania, Croatia, and Slovenia, support for communist ideals created opportunities for establishing institutions of welfare and social service (Waaldijk, 2011).

In the aftermath of the Cold War, Western social welfare practices served as ideological tools in showing the humane side of capitalism (Lorenz, 2008). The development of social work in Nicaragua exemplifies this. The US provided aid and introduced social policies in Nicaragua in a bid to stem the fomenting of revolutions following the Cuban revolutionaries' victories of 1959 (Kreitzer & Wilson, 2010). Then, in the 1970s and early 1980s, social workers came under attack because the new government viewed them as aides of the old regime. This affected and undermined social work education, resulting in a hold on new student admissions for social work training and education (Kreitzer & Wilson, 2010).

In other places, despotic administrations caused the closure of institutions committed to social work education and practice. For some time, social work was excluded from academic study for political reasons in countries such as Chile, Spain, and Hungary (Weiss-Gal & Welbourne, 2008).

Social Work's Human Rights Activism

Even in its early days, the social work profession focused on a diversity of issues, not just the provision of relief to the poor. The pioneers of social work such as Jane Addams, Sophonisba Breckinridge, Julia Lathrop, and Grace Abbott participated in human rights movements too (Healy, 2008). In the UK, Eglantyne Jebb shifted focus from the Charity Organization Society to children's rights. She penned the first Declaration of the Rights of the Child in 1923, later taken by the League of Nations as the Declaration of Geneva in 1924 (Healy, 2008). Alice Salomon, founder of social work in Germany, also participated in human rights activities, notably in women's rights (Healy, 2008). Some of these pioneers influenced state policies on social welfare (Abrams & Curran, 2004).

Many believe that, regardless of the differences that exist among countries, they all face the same social problems. These problems include aging populations, migration issues, and populations with low socio-economic status (Hendriks, Kloppenburg, Gevorgianiene & Jakutiene, 2008; Hines, Cohen, Tran, Lee, & Van Phu, 2010).

Standards for Social Work Practice

The social work profession's standards streamline practice and serve to protect clients (NASW, 2008; Sewpaul & Jones, 2005). However, these standards vary widely throughout the world. While many countries require registration or certification of social workers, others do not. Whereas social workers' registration in the UK is mandatory, in New Zealand it is non-binding. In the UK practitioners' registration is a prerequisite for practice and makes one eligible to use the title of social worker. Some countries have laws which reinforce social workers' status and professional education. For example in Scotland, use of the "social worker" title prior to registration is a crime (Orme & Rennie, 2006). What constitutes a social worker in different countries varies significantly. Some countries require a Bachelor's degree in social work, while others require no degree at all. For example, in Sweden, Hungary, and India, there are no licensing procedures for social workers and no legislative instruments guarding the use of the title "social worker."

Conclusion

The problems social workers handle are prevalent across the globe. Thus, there is a need for social workers with the skills and competencies to work with diverse populations. Social workers need to be able to adapt their training and education to infuse perspectives from other cultures into their local settings (Hendriks et al., 2008). Social work practices can be learned from other cultures and modified to match the needs of a practitioner's local population (Ashencaen Crabtree, 2008). The long-standing tradition of Western social work has a great deal of experience to offer budding social work professions around the world. However, Western social work has as much to learn from other cultures as to impart to them (Hutchings & Taylor, 2007). This learning can inspire and enhance social work practice nationally and locally (Hendriks et al., 2008). The development of theoretical and practice models to suit the areas and localities where workers practice should take into account important cultural realities and sensitivities (Dominelli, 2010).

Our book aims to educate social work practitioners around the world and address the questions: What is local about social work? What is specific about social work to different countries and contexts? What is the same in social work practice the world over? We hope our attempts to answer these questions here will inspire continued dialogue on this topic wherever you are.

Taking a practical hands-on approach, this text includes a dedicated section for classroom use, with discussion questions, classroom exercises, and additional cases for your own analysis. It will be particularly useful to BSW and MSW students taking courses in international social work, practice, social welfare, and human behaviour. Eight additional case studies and 16 analyses from social workers in various countries are available online at http://www.routledge.com/books/details/9780415783668/

References

Abrams, L. & Curran, L. (2004). Between women: Gender and social work in historical perspective. *Social Service Review, 78(3)*, 429–447.

Al-Krenawi, A. (1999). "Social workers practicing in their non-western home communities: Overcoming conflict between professional and cultural values." *Families in Society*, 80, 488–95.

Ashencaen Crabtree, S. (2008). "Dilemmas in international social work education in the United Arab Emirates: Islam, localization and social need." *Social Work Education*, 27, 536–48.

Austin, D. M. (1983). "The Flexner myth and the history of social work." *Social Service Review*, 57, 357–77.

Crafts, N., & Fearon, P. (2010). "Lessons from the 1930s Great Depression." *Oxford Review of Economic Policy*, 26, 285–317.

Dominelli, L. (2010). "Globalization, contemporary challenges and social work practice." *International Social Work*, 53, 599–612.

Dyeson, T. (2004). "Social work update. Social work licensure: A brief history and description." *Home Health Care Management & Practice*, 16, 408–11.

Garvin C. D. and Tropman J. E. (1998). *Social work in contemporary society, second edition*. Allyn and Bacon.

Graham, J. R. (2005). "Religion." In F. J. Turner (Ed.). Encyclopedia of Canadian Social Work (pp. 320–22). Ontario: Wilfrid Laurier University Press

Graham, J. R., Hazarika, S., & Narasimhan, K. (2011). "Financial distress in the Great Depression." *Financial Management*, 40, 821–44.

Gray, M., & Fook, J. (2004). "The quest for a universal social work: Some issues and implications." *Social Work Education*, 23, 625–44.

Hare, I. (2004). "Defining social work for the 21st century: The international federation of social workers' revised definition of social work." *International Social Work*, 47, 407–24.

Healy, L. (2008). "Exploring the history of social work as a human rights profession." *International Social Work*, 51, 735–48.

Healy, L., and Thomas, R. (2007). "International social work: A retrospective in the 50th year." *International Social Work*, 50, 581–96.

Hendriks, P., Kloppenburg, R., Gevorgianiene, V., & Jakutiene, V. (2008). "Cross-national social work case analysis: Learning from international experience within an electronic environment." *European Journal of Social Work*, 11, 383–96.

Herrick J. M. (2005). "Settlement houses (United States)." In J. M. Herrick and P. H. Stuart (Eds.). *Encyclopedia of social welfare history in North America* (pp. 384–86). California: Sage Publications, Inc.

Hines, A. M., Cohen, E., Tran, T., Lee, P., & Van Phu, L. (2010). "The development of social work in Vietnam: The role of international collaboration." *Social Work Education*, 29, 910–22.

Hugman, R. (1996). "Professionalization in social work: The challenge of diversity." *International Social Work*, 39: 131–47.

Hugman, R., Moosa-Mitha, M., & Moyo, O. (2010). "Towards a borderless social work: Reconsidering notions of international social work." *International Social Work*, 53 (5), 629–43.

Hutchings, A., & Taylor, I. (2007). "Defining the profession? Exploring an international definition of social work in the China context." *International Journal of Social Welfare*, 16, 382–90.

International Federation of Social Workers (IFSW) (2000) "Definition of social work. General Meeting Montréal, Québec, Canada." Retrieved from http://www.ifsw.org/f38000138.html

Jacques, G. (2011). "Echoes of a primal scream: AIDS and fostering in Botswana." *The Social Work Practitioner-Researcher/Die Maatskaplikewerk Navorser-Praktisyn*, 23 (2), 154–70.

Kreitzer, L., & Wilson, M. (2010). "Shifting perspectives on international alliances in social work: Lessons from Ghana and Nicaragua." *International Social Work*, 53, 701–19

Kohs, S. C., (1966). *The roots of social work*. New York: Associations Press.

Jennissen, T., & Lundy, C. (2005). Social work profession (Canada). In J. M. Herrick and P. H. Stuart (Eds.). *Encyclopedia of social welfare history in North America* (pp. 384–86). California: Sage Publications, Inc.

Lorenz, W. (2008). "Towards a European model of social work." *Australian Social Work*, 61, 7–24.

Lough, B. J. (2009). "Curricular blueprinting: The relevance of American social work education for international students." *Social Work Education*, 28 (7), 792–802.

Markus, H., & Kitayama, S. (1991). "Culture and the self: Implications for cognition, emotion, and motivation." *Psychological Review*, 98, 224–53.

McPhail, B. A. (2004). "Setting the record straight: Social work is not a female-dominated profession." *Social Work*, 49, 323–26.

Moldovan, V., & Moyo, O. (2007). Contradictions in the ideologies of helping: Examples from Zimbabwe and Moldova. *International Social Work*, 50, 461–472.

Mwansa, L. (2011). "Social work education in Africa: Whence and whither?" *Social Work Education*, 30, 4–16.

National Association of Social Workers (NASW). (2008). "Preamble to the code of ethics." Retrieved from http://www.socialworkers.org/pubs/code/code. asp

Oanh, N. (2002). "Historical development and characteristics of social work in today's Vietnam." *International Journal of Social Welfare*, 11, 84–91.

Orme, J., & Rennie, G. (2006). "The role of registration in ensuring ethical practice." *International Social Work*, 49, 333–344.

Sewpaul, V., & Jones, D. (2005). Global standards for the education and training of the social work profession. *International Journal of Social Welfare*, 14 (3), 218–230.

Soliman, H., & Elmegied, H. (2010). "The Challenges of modernization of social work education in developing countries: The case of Egypt." *International Social Work*, 53, 101–14.

Stuart, P. H. (2005). "Social work profession (Canada)". In J. M. Herrick and P. H. Stuart (Eds.), *Encyclopedia of social welfare history in North America* (pp. 384–86). California: Sage Publications, Inc.

Waaldijk, B. (2011). "Social work between oppression and emancipation histories of discomfort and inspiration in Europe." *Social Work & Society International Online Journal*, 9, 1–16. Retrieved from http://www.socwork.net/sws/article/view/272/607

Webb, S. (2007). "The comfort of strangers: social work, modernity and late Victorian England – part II." *European Journal of Social Work*, 10, 193–207.

Wedemeyer, J. M., & Moore, P. (1966). "The American welfare system." *California Law Review*, 54, 326–56.

Weiss, I., Spiro, S., Sherer, M. & Korin-Langer, N. (2004). "Social work in Israel: Professional characteristics in an international comparative perspective." *International Journal of Social Welfare*, 13, 287–96.

Weiss-Gal, I., & Welbourne, P. (2008). "The professionalisation of social work: A cross-national exploration." *International Journal of Social Welfare*, 17, 281–90.

Xu, Q. (2006). "Defining international social work: A social service agency perspective." *International Social Work*, 49, 679–92.

<table>
<tr><td>2</td><td># Child Welfare</td></tr>
</table>

Child Welfare

By Gloria Jacques

Child welfare is a dominant issue of public concern around the world. Some of the major issues in this arena include those surrounding physical, emotional, psychological or sexual child abuse and neglect. Unfortunately, there is no single standard for what constitutes abuse or neglect at the global level. Certain acts perceived to have adverse social and health implications in the development of children in certain societies may be normative in others. Thus the conceptualization of child abuse and neglect, its scope and causes, and the forms in which these issues are manifested vary within and across cultures making it difficult to pronounce judgment on what sets of child rearing practices are appropriate and acceptable in different countries. Furthermore in various epochs of human existence, these practices have differed in relation to acceptability (Gelles, 2007). The information in the case studies and analyses in this chapter reflects these differing definitions and situations.

Case study #1

Three Children in a Home are Neglected

BY RUTH GERRITSEN-McKANE FROM THE US

It was 10:30 in the evening when Sarah, age six, Jonathan, age four, and Annie, age three, started out on their adventure to their favorite place to play. Sparsely dressed, the three walked away from their house. Walking along a busy highway the children became frightened by the traffic and so, huddling together, cold and tired, they sat down on the sidewalk. Sarah sat between Jonathan and Annie with her arms wrapped around them trying to keep them warm. It was close to midnight when one of the drivers on the highway noticed the children. He pulled over and contacted the local police department. Concerned that he might scare the children if he approached them, he stayed a distance away that would permit him to keep an eye on them until the police arrived.

At 12:30 in the morning a police officer and child protection worker were on the scene. The children were placed in the back of a patrol car and wrapped in a large blanket. The child protection worker began to question the children as to what their names were, where they were headed, where they lived, and whether there was anyone at home looking after them. Sarah quietly introduced herself and her brother and sister. She explained that they were on their way to a playground "just down the street." The child protection worker asked why they were going out to play so late. Jonathan responded, "We didn't get to play today; we had to stay in the house while mommy and daddy went out. When daddy got home and lay down we asked if we could play and he said yes." "Was your mom home?" the child protection worker asked. Sarah responded, "Nope, she will come home in the morning, that's when she comes home." "So do you know how to get home?" the police officer asked. "Yup, just that way," Jonathan replied. Tucked into the back seat of the patrol car, the officer drove in the direction Jonathan pointed and the case worker followed behind. The police officer called for additional officers to help and the case worker made a call to her supervisor.

Three Children in a Home are Neglected: A Social Worker from Ghana Responds

BY KWADWO OFORI-DUA

Prevalence and Incidence

Child abuse is on the increase throughout Ghana. Media reports and records of the Department of Social Welfare (DSW) in the Ashanti region suggest that there has also been an increase in the number of child neglect cases. In 2009, the number of neglected children recorded by the Department stood at 1,367. This figure went up to 1,761 in 2010 (DSW Archives, n.d.). Likewise the Brong-Ahafo office of the Domestic Violence and Victim Support Unit (DOVVSU) of the Ghana Police Service recorded, between January and September 2010, 665 cases of child non-maintenance as compared to 499 cases for the same period the previous year (DOVVSU, 2010).

The statistics are alarming, but represent only the tip of the iceberg, with most cases, especially those of neglect and sexual and emotional abuse, going unreported. In many settings, however, the line between deliberate child neglect and that which is caused by ignorance or lack of alternatives may be difficult to draw.

Country Policies

There is a general consensus in social work that the social services in any country are related to the economic development of that country, the nature of the political system, the overall structure of the society, and traditional methods of meeting social needs in that country. The transition from a strong traditional society through the stages of colonial rule to the period of political independence has had a significant impact on the field of social work in Ghana. This history determines what it is, why it is necessary, and the character and orientation of social welfare professionals.

Technically, there were no social workers in traditional Ghanaian society. This lack does not mean that there were no social problems. People in all societies have always had problems related to issues such as deprivation, want, deviance, and death. In traditional Ghana, these problems were not the province of a specialized cadre of workers. They were, however, addressed by the social groups to which a person belonged, most particularly the family, lineage or community. This orientation of group responsibility, being "my brother's keeper" or concern for one another, was the value of traditional African societies.

Currently, in Ghana, social services are mainly provided by the DSW, (under the umbrella of the Ministry of Employment and Social Welfare) and a number of non-governmental organizations (NGOs). Social workers are found in health care settings, correctional centers, destitute infirmaries, and residential centers for children in need of care. They render services in community care and children's rights and protection, and assist the DOVVSU of the Ghana Police Service in handling domestic violence and abuse cases.

Policies and laws to protect the rights and interests of children include the Children's Act of 1998 and the Child Rights Regulation of 2002. The Children's Act defines a child as any person below the age of 18 and describes the basic rights of the child, supports family tribunals, and sets rules governing parental duty, custody, labor, apprenticeship, care, and protection so that children develop to their full potential. The best interests of a child are to be paramount in any matter concerning them and every parent is, therefore, duty bound to ensure the well-being of their children including protection from neglect.

The Early Childhood and Development Policy (2006) also provides for the full protection, nurturing, and development of children by parents and society as a whole. In addition, the Legal Aid Scheme Act of 1997 states that children must be treated with the utmost care in relation to their protection, growth, and development. The enforcement of these laws and policies is entrusted to several public institutions. These include the Commission on Children (GNCC), the DSW, and the DOVVSU of the Ghana Police Service.

A Social Worker Responds

One of the ethical considerations of professional social work is to help people in need and to address social problems (National Association of Social Workers [NASW], 1999) irrespective of their age, color, creed, and race (including children who are particularly vulnerable). With regard to the current case, the social worker would first secure the safety of the minors and attend to their immediate needs, especially involving their evacuation to a safe place if necessary. The worker would then make the necessary arrangements to have their health status checked by medical personnel and ensure the provision of needed health care and support, especially the availability of adequate and appropriate nutrition. The social worker would liaise with the police and the DSW to ensure that the children have decent accommodation and appropriate and adequate clothing to keep them warm since they were sparsely dressed in a cold climate when found. The worker would then ensure their safety and protection with their parents or guardians in their own home (if possible) and, if not, secure temporary accommodation. In the Ghanaian context, this arrangement would be made in conjunction with the police and officials of the DSW.

After securing the safety and attending to the immediate needs of the children, the social worker would proceed to prepare a social history and assessment report for the benefit of other professionals who may be involved in the case. The report would enable the worker and other professionals to obtain a deeper understanding of the children and their social environment (family, community, and school) and how these affect their well-being. In preparing the report, the social worker would first interview the children and corroborate information obtained from them through visiting their families, neighborhood, and schools to personally observe environmental factors. These data would be used to formulate an intervention strategy or recommendations for meeting the children's needs.

Since they are all minors, the worker would have to develop intervention strategies with appropriate agencies and institutions concerned with the welfare and development of children so that each could play a role in ensuring their welfare. A committee made up of officials of the DSW, Ghana Police Service, Ghana Education Service, Ministry of Women and Children Affairs, Attorney General's Office, and a social worker would be formed to assess the problem and formulate intervention plans. If it is established that the safety and welfare of the children cannot be guaranteed under the care of their parents or guardians, the state may consider the option of taking custody of the children. However, if the evidence on the ground suggests that their well-being would best be served by leaving them with their parents, then the latter would be compelled to ensure proper care and supervision of the children by signing an undertaking to that effect.

The committee's decisions would be implemented in the best interests of the children and the social worker would be the coordinator of all activities of the implementing agencies. Not only would he/she ensure that the children's human rights are upheld but he/she would also ascertain that all services would facilitate the children's growth and development. The social worker would have to monitor their progress in school, their health status, and their general well-being. The worker will also liaise with both governmental and non-governmental agencies to ensure that the children do not lack anything relevant to their welfare and development.

If the results are encouraging, the worker will sustain the intervention. On the other hand, if the best interests of the children are not being served, he/she has to review the strategies in consultation with appropriate agencies and institutions.

Three Children in a Home are Neglected: A Social Worker from Botswana Responds

BY TOBOKANE MANTHAI

Prevalence and Incidence

Child neglect is not a new issue for Botswana. However, there is very limited information on prevalence and incidence, which is attributed to closed family and community ties resulting in most cases of child neglect and abuse being unreported or undocumented. According to Ruiz-Casares and Heymann (2009), in one-half of the families in Botswana children are left at home alone on a regular or occasional basis. They further note that

52 per cent of families leave children home alone and rely on other children to help with child care due to limited support networks in urban areas. This situation may result in unsafe child care arrangements and limited parental involvement, and expose children to injuries and other risks as discussed in the case study.

Country Policies

Tswana society's way of life has been historically agricultural and societal values emphasize division of labor, designated forms of assistance, and attending to the needs of the family. Women have the domestic responsibility to breed, nurture, and take care of children, whilst men spend most of their time providing for the family through agricultural or formal employment.

Botswana has seen various developments in the last two decades on laws in education, child welfare, and alternative care for young people. However, recent socio-economic and political developments in education and employment have influenced gender roles to the extent that men no longer solely identify with provision for the family and growing numbers are also involved in the daily nurturing of children.

Migration is a large factor in Botswana. Many families and their young children have migrated from rural to urban areas for better access to education, shelter, employment, and health care. Children are generally seen as valuable resources of the entire family, government, and society. The above factors have influenced family types and have caused family structures to transition from extended to nuclear, single-headed, or blended families.

The present pattern of employed women and possible involvement of fathers in the nurturing of children born inside or outside of marriage has affected the traditional practice of sending children to maternal grand-mothers for fostering. Children live with parents in towns and cities and there is usually limited access to child care. This phenomenon has led to child abuse and neglect.

Botswana has several policies in place to respond to issues affecting children. These include: the National Plan of Action (NPA) for Children 2006–2016, which is used to inform programs for children in the areas of education and training, health and nutrition, children and HIV and AIDS, sport and recreation, child protection, environment and safety, and policy and legislation. The 1981 Children's Act was amended in 2009 in conformity with the United Nations Convention on the Rights of the Child (1989), and it includes protection of children in exceptionally difficult circumstances. In addition, the development of Children in Need of Care

Regulations in 2005 defines statutory fostering processes and procedures, and these are currently (2012) being finalized in relation to the 2009 Children's Act. The Convention on the Rights of the Child assumes overall responsibility for the coordination of policies relating to children or for monitoring the implementation of children's rights and welfare issues.

A Social Worker Responds

Child neglect in this case presents as a pattern of failing to provide for children's basic needs in the form of clothing, hygiene, supervision, and safety. Sara, being the older child, might not show outward signs of neglect. She presents a competent face to the outside world, even taking on the role of the parent by having her arms around her two siblings to protect them. It is obvious that these three neglected children are not getting their physical and emotional needs met.

Professional social work practice in Botswana utilizes a multifaceted approach that involves child welfare, social welfare, and community development services to meet the needs of children and their families. Integration of various approaches is required to help families with child abuse and/or neglect issues to change their perspective and accomplish constructive goals. Approaches and theories utilized by social workers include: community systems and resources; cognitive-behavioral or rational-emotive theories; task-centered practice; family therapy; and an eclectic mode of intervention. Social workers attempt to maintain nonjudgmental attitudes and encourage family involvement, and have no preconceived notions about a family's motivation. Most families in Botswana are open to change for the better, especially if the change is aimed at protecting their children rather than removing their children from them, although some are struggling with the demands placed upon them by AIDS and orphanhood.

Social workers adopt a team approach through which team members use their varied knowledge and expertise to assess and manage the problems of child abuse and neglect from the vantage point of their different perspectives. Examples here include state, local authority, and NGOs' input. Team members work with the family during the initial response, developing a brief treatment plan with specific strategies to foster the issues' resolution and healthy family functioning. It is the responsibility of the social worker to consult with other members and related professionals to ensure that assessment, planning, and intervention techniques incorporate the full team's knowledge and experience, and are responsive to the needs of the parents and children by enabling them to choose problem-solving strategies that restore their sense of well-being and ability to cope.

The social worker also helps to provide stability and consistent support for two families in need of child care services by guiding them to appropriate organizations such as Childline Botswana. The worker collaborates with the parents to assess available support from family, friends, and neighbors willing to offer help during their absence. The social worker works with the couple to assess the applicability and feasibility of roles and responsibilities, for example, by adopting the family-treatment approach that focuses on failures of role performance as a parent or spouse, and considers role confusion and role reversal to be present in child neglect and abuse cases.

On a regular basis, children in Botswana spend a variable amount of time under the supervision of other caregivers in formal and informal settings, and a substantial number provide unsupervised self- or sibling care for varying periods of time. In many instances, children like Sara are expected to display greater maturity and assume a greater sense of responsibility in caring for their siblings. This expectation is common in child- or youth-headed households, which are mostly a result of orphanhood due to loss of parents to AIDS. The absence of adults in the household leaves children unsupervised meaning higher exposure to accidents and injuries, increased risky and antisocial behavior (for example, substance use and delinquency), poorer school performance (or non-attendance), and negative developmental outcomes. Neglected children may benefit from individual counseling and other forms of therapy but this is not always readily available. In urban areas, therapy is more accessible than in villages and remote locations. Furthermore, the social worker needs to be watchful of delinquent behavior or acting out by survivors of child abuse and neglect. It is important for the worker to work with children to manage emotions and exercise some level of control in their lives as they mature or to consider placement with organizations such as Mpule Kwelagobe residential care facility and Childline Botswana's place of safety.

Batswana parents tend to trust young and old domestic helpers with the lives of their children. Stories have been published in the media about acts of physical, sexual, and emotional abuse and neglect perpetrated by such caregivers. The reported incidents include the suffocation, burning, starving, pinching, beating, and bruising, as well as the trafficking of children by their caregivers. These experiences have led to diminished trust of caregivers and parents having to be more careful about whom they choose as care providers.

Ideally, social workers work with the families to devise means of ensuring child safety and security in their absence. Continuous assessment and monitoring of the family is maintained. If child abuse and neglect persists, the social worker takes the case before the Children's Court and recommends removal of the child to a place of safety. This place could be residential care provided, on a limited scale, by the state or non-governmental organizations, or customary care in kinship systems organized by local authority social workers. Although statutory foster care is provided for in the legislation and many social workers have been specifically trained for this program, it is still in the process of implementation.

Customary or statutory foster care or adoption should attempt to prevent separation of siblings as this has been observed to impact children negatively. Some children have been reported to commit suicide or roam the streets after placement. It is the social worker's responsibility to ensure that children are appropriately placed and adapt positively to their new environment. If child neglect is due to the parents' negligent behavior, the social worker works with parents to help them learn what is age appropriate (what Sara is capable and not capable of handling) and to develop their own parenting skills with regard to appropriate discipline and the setting of clear boundaries for children. The social worker employs cognitive behavioral therapies to help parents address their irrational beliefs, thoughts, and behaviors that lead to child neglect.

Case study #2

Possible Child Abuse

BY KWAKU OSEI-HWEDIE & MORENA J. RANKOPO FROM BOTSWANA

Lerato, a 40-year-old mother of four, lives with her 52-year-old husband, Kagiso, and her 60-year-old mother, Gaone. Both Gaone and Kagiso are retired civil servants while Lerato is a clerk for an insurance company. The oldest of Lerato and Kagiso's four children is Moshe who is a 16-year-old student at a secondary school. The other children are aged 12, ten and seven, respectively, and are still in primary school.

Lerato's older sister, Malebogo, who is 54 years old, lives two houses away from her. Lerato became ill and was hospitalized but the hospital could not diagnose any specific ailment suggesting that the problem might be psycho-social. Upon hearing this, Malebogo went to the social worker and said that the help needed by her sister was not medical. She informed the social worker that it is not only her sister, but everybody in the household that needs help.

She said that Lerato is sexually involved with her 16-year-old son, while her husband is sexually involved with his mother-in-law. She was concerned that the younger children might be aware of what is happening among the older family members. She said she was afraid that the younger children risked being forced into the network of familial sexual abuse. Malebogo did not want her sister to know that she had spoken to the social worker but was prepared to help in any way she could in providing support to family members. She appeared to be extremely hostile towards her brother-in-law which was understandable. However, the social worker detected an element of jealousy in Malebogo's attitude towards her sister.

Possible Child Abuse: A Social Worker from India Responds

BY HENA JOHN-FISK

Prevalence and Incidence

In India, data on incidence and prevalence of child sexual abuse is incomplete because most of the children who face sexual abuse do not report the traumatic event due to the belief in Indian society that sexual abuse does not happen, or if it happens it should be kept secret. The laws do not bring speedy justice to these survivors of abuse, another factor which also leads to a low incidence of reporting. In India, each law dealing with children defines the age of a child differently, which makes it difficult and confusing to report the abuse. In addition, the existing laws do not cover crimes against children. Due to the above reasons, there was a lack of a national database on child sexual abuse until recently when the Indian Government created the Ministry of Women and Child Development (MWCD) to look into issues surrounding child protection. The MWCD in collaboration with UNICEF, save the children, and other national and local NGOs in 13 states conducted a nationwide study involving 12,447 children, 2,324 young adults, and 2,449 stakeholders. The study found that 5–12 year olds are at the highest risk of abuse and exploitation, with 53.22 per cent reporting having faced one or more forms of sexual abuse. Andhra Pradesh, Assam, Bihar and Delhi provinces reported the highest percentage of sexual abuse among both boys and girls as well as the highest incidence of sexual assault (MWCD, 2007). Furthermore, 21.9 per cent of child participants reported facing severe forms of sexual abuse, 50.7 per cent reported other types of sexual abuse, and 5.6 per cent reported being sexually assaulted. Children who are homeless, at work, or in institutional care reported high incidences of sexual assault. Fifty per cent of these abuse cases were by people who knew the child or were in a position of trust and responsibility (MWCD, 2007). Apart from this study, leading daily newspapers report more than two to three incidences of minor rape or sexual abuse of girl children. Cases of male child rape and sexual abuse are still unknown due to a failure to report such incidents.

Country Policies

Indian society considers children an integral part of the family unit and not as individuals with specific rights. The Indian constitution has issued certain fundamental rights to children which are needs- and not rights-based. It was not until recently that the Indian Government started looking at protection as an aspect of a child's right. In this regard, MWCD was created to specifically address child protection issues. The MWCD then presented the Offences against Children (Prevention) Bill, but due to a lack of data on child sexual abuse this bill was not passed. Thus there is still no single universal law to protect children from sexual abuse in India. However, there are a few laws which address the issue of child sexual abuse although they have their limitations. For instance, every child-related law defines the age of a child differently, which makes it difficult and confusing to report abuse. Child sexual abuse is addressed in the Indian Penal Code (IPC), Juvenile Justice Act (2000), and the Information Technology Act (2000), but there is no specific law that can punish pedophiles or compensate the victims of such events. The IPC does not include males as rape victims.

A Social Worker Responds

Due to a lack of specific child abuse laws it is very difficult to obtain justice for the survivors of child sexual abuse. The case at hand would be addressed in two different ways dependent upon the professional to whom Malebogo has reported the situation. If it was a medical social worker in a hospital then it would be addressed in the following manner. After talking to Malebogo, the social worker would prepare an intake sheet and write down all the necessary information. Then the social worker would call the Childline India Foundation, which provides protection to all children and has a 24-hour helpline service for children in distress. The social worker would refer the children to the Foundation for legal procedures and rehabilitation processes.

Childline would file a First Information Report (FIR) of sexual abuse of Moshe to the police under sections 375, 376, and 377 of the IPC. According to Section 375, a man is said to commit "rape" when he has sexual intercourse with a woman or girl-child against her will or consent, with her consent by putting her in a life-threatening situation or on the pretext of being her husband. Section 376 defines the punishment for rape as imprisonment for seven years, but it could be for a term that may extend to ten years or for life. Section 377 of the IPC (2007 amendment) criminalizes all non-consensual penile, non-vaginal sex, and penile non-vaginal sex involving minors (Mitta & Singh, 2009). The punishments for sexual abuse offenders are the same as for rape. It would be hard to prosecute Lerato under these laws since they do not define rape or abuse of a male child by a woman. Even with these loopholes, Lerato could still be arrested and tried for sexual abuse under the Indian judicial system. She could get bail, since sexual abuse is a non-cognitive offense, and the court could also decide to take custody of her children. The court could give the custody of the children to Kagiso, the father of the children. Even though Kagiso has a sexual relationship with Gaone (the grandmother of his children), the court could still give custody to him as his relationship with Gaone would not be considered a crime, although due to this relationship Lerato could get a divorce from Kagiso.

Additionally, Childline would take Moshe and the other children to the Child Welfare Committee (CWC) because, under the Juvenile Justice Act (2000), they are in need of care and protection. The CWC would refer all the children to boarding homes which are shelters where a child stays until the age of 18, pursues his/her education, and receives psychosocial intervention. All four siblings would preferably be kept in the same, or nearby, boarding homes where they would receive counseling. If the court gives custody to the father, then the CWC could order psychosocial intervention for the children in his care. Along with this, the CWC could ask the social workers to conduct home visits, provide psychosocial intervention to the family, and report on the situation to the CWS.

Psychosocial intervention at the boarding school or the NGO would be similar. The social worker could meet Moshe and the other three siblings, and build rapport with them after which they would be informed about counseling sessions in line with their maturity and understanding of the situation. They would also be informed about the objectives and details of the intervention. Each child would receive individual and group interventions. The children would then be referred to a counselor within the organization. The counselor would build rapport with each child and explain to them the counseling process and its objectives.

In this section, we will focus on Moshe's counseling sessions. It could take several sessions before he might start talking about the abuse. After finding out about the traumatic events, the counselor might also encourage Moshe to address his feelings towards the event (such as guilt and self-hate) and explore his academic life. The counselor might work with Moshe's personality issues, such as becoming an introvert or getting involved in other sexual relations out of anger towards his mother. The counselor would also discuss with Moshe his feelings about the legal aspect of the situation and rehabilitation, such as how he feels, and what his concerns are about staying with his family/father or in a government shelter (boarding home).

Along with Moshe's counseling, his other three siblings will receive psychosocial intervention. Play therapy could be used to understand if these children have been abused themselves, if they are aware of Moshe's situation or their father's relationship with their grandmother, and how to address these issues. These children would receive individual and group counseling with each other and with Moshe too.

Apart from these sessions the counselor could have a joint session with the couple (Lerato and Kagiso), a session with the parents and the children, and one with the grandmother (Gaone). These sessions would revolve around the impact and consequences of their relationship on their children's mental state, education, personality, and life. The social worker may contact Lerato and ask her if she would like to talk about her feelings concerning the situation. Only if she agrees will the social worker listen to her story and ask about her children, husband, and the sexual abuse of Moshe. The social worker would then inquire whether she would want to be part of the psychosocial intervention process together with her family and refer her if she agrees. After all the sessions the counselor would submit a report to the social worker.

If Malebogo had reported this case to a social worker in an NGO, there would be no contact made with Childline. The social worker would first talk to Moshe and his siblings. The NGO would file the FIR with the police and refer all the children to the CWC, and similar legal processes, counseling, and rehabilitation procedures would be followed.

Possible Child Abuse: A Social Worker from Finland Responds

BY RIITA VÄÄNÄNEN, RIITA VORNANEN, PIRJO PÖLKKI, & JUHA HÄMÄLÄINEN

Prevalence and Incidence

The Child Welfare Act (2007) considers that a person under the age of 18 years is a child. Sexual abuse is defined either as intercourse or any other kind of sexual act with a child under the age of 16. According to Finnish criminal law, a person who is the parent of a 16- to 17-year-old adolescent or is living in the same household as that child, commits a crime if he or she has intercourse with the child or behaves in a sexual way that is harmful to the child.

Violence against children and children's sexual abuse is a hidden problem, the prevalence of which is very difficult to evaluate (see Hélie, Clément & Larrivée, 2003). In Finland, the prevalence of violence against children and child abuse has been studied mainly in two ways: by researching the victimization of children and by studying statistics. However, according to Humppi and Ellonen (2010), statistics give information about detected cases, not the prevalence of the problem. This discrepancy has been observed by comparing the statistics and victimization numbers in surveys. Here we focus both on the statistics for Finland and studies on the prevalence of child abuse, especially sexual abuse. During recent decades, police statistics in Finland show that the number of child sexual abuse cases has increased (Niemi 2007; Niemi, 2010; Hinkkanen, 2009), although, in 2009, the number had begun to decrease (Niemi, 2010). The previous increase does not necessarily mean that child abuse is more prevalent; instead the readiness to speak out against it has grown and the monitoring of cases by the authorities has become more effective.

Surveys carried out in Finland show changing trends in the prevalence of child abuse. In 1988, 13 per cent of 15-year-old children reported sexual experiences with partners at least five years older than themselves (Sariola, 1988), whereas in 2008 the number of teenagers reporting this was 8 per cent (Ellonen, Kääriäinen, Salmi, & Sariola, 2008). On the other hand, the number of negative experiences had increased as had sexual experiences with adult strangers and, because of the development of information technology, sexual harassment on the internet was quite common. Currently, there is evidence of increasing internet-based sexual abuse (Niemi, 2007; Ellonen et al., 2008; Niemi 2010; Ministry of Social Affairs and Health, 2009) and effective preventive measures are needed to help children avoid risks in this regard.

According to the 2008 survey, the incidence of familial sexual abuse had decreased over a 20-year period. Nordic countries have cooperated in developing a common framework for youth surveys in the areas of sexual abuse and exposure to violence (Helweg-Larsen, 2009). However, the different statistics and measures of surveys produce different rates of prevalence and thus the exact extent of this phenomenon is unknown.

Country Policies

Since the 1960s, Finnish society has adhered to the Nordic model of social welfare. The welfare system is based on the idea of social citizenship, according to which citizens have broad social rights and duties. National insurance is relatively comprehensive in terms of health insurance, unemployment benefits, retirement pensions, and other benefits. Characteristics of this social welfare model are highly developed services for children and families (Esping-Andersen, 2002). Social work has been developed as part of this Nordic welfare system and it is an important professional instrument in the socio-political infrastructure.

The Child Welfare Act (417/2007) obligates every municipality in Finland to provide child welfare services. The basic principles of child welfare are the same as those in the UN Convention on the Rights of the Child, and Finland is committed to the European Convention for the Protection of Human Rights (European Court, 2010). Child welfare social work is built on the principle of supporting both family life and parents in the task of raising their children.

Efforts have been made to develop cooperation and expertise in the prevention and treatment of violence, which means that municipalities, inter-municipal cooperation, and hospital districts must have well-functioning practices to intervene when children are subjected to violence (Nursing Research Foundation, 2008.) There is also a strong emphasis on awareness and identifying the early signs of violence, especially in basic services that have access to and meet with all families and children. Examples of such services are day care facilities, baby clinics, and schools. There are different levels of policies and procedures in the prevention and treatment of sexual abuse. A need for general crime prevention exists; in addition, the prevention of child abuse by means of family policy and social and health services is also necessary. General measures against increasingly prevalent internet-based risks may also prevent crimes against children.

In 1989, Finland ratified the Convention on the Rights of the Child and committed to protect children against all forms of sexual abuse (Article 34). In 2007, Finland also signed the Council of Europe's Convention on the Protection of Children against Sexual Exploitation and Sexual Abuse, and evaluated its national policy and legislation in the light of that convention. One example is the Finnish Government's Internal Security Program (Ministry of the Interior, 2008) which, by means of safety skills education, aims at instructing children on how to protect themselves against potential and actual sexual abuse through electronic interactive media.

In 2008, the Ministry of Social Affairs and Health set up a committee to evaluate the practices in assessing and investigating problems in this area.

This evaluation was realized in the form of multi-professional cooperation between the police, the prosecuting attorney and the social and health care sector (Ministry of Social Affairs and Health, 2009). The Finnish Medical Society developed evidence-based guidelines for investigation of the sexual abuse of a child (Current Care Summary, 2006). A clinical practice guideline was also introduced by the Nursing Research Foundation (2008) for the early detection of child maltreatment.

Child abuse within a family has been relatively hidden, and for a fairly long time it was seen as the family's own internal matter and not an issue of public concern. However, perceptions of this issue have changed. The Child Welfare Act (417/2007) requires that the municipal body responsible for social services be notified if it becomes apparent that there is a necessity to investigate a case on account of the child's need for care, circumstances endangering the child's development or the child's behavior (Section 25).

In Finland, an inquiry into sexual abuse is a criminal inquiry and the main responsibility lies with the police organization. The police will decide what measures are needed and make letters of request to the health care services for the investigation. Investigations in health care have been funded by the state since 2009. Since the sexual abuse of minors is a very sensitive phenomenon, the process in Finland is very strictly guided by both legal and practical guidelines. Inquiries are centralized in the departments of child and adolescent psychiatry in university hospitals (Government Bill for the Act 126/2008; Act on organizing the investigation of sexual crimes against children no. 1009/2008). The latest Child Welfare Act (417/2007) clearly specifies a social worker's qualification requirements on the basis of tasks and defines a social worker's eligibility to deal with core child and family-specific statutory child protection responsibilities and the exercise of public authority. They have autonomy with regard to professional decision-making, but there is also a strong emphasis on multi-professional cooperation.

A Social Worker Responds

In Finland, the process for handling this type of case would begin with a preliminary investigation by a child welfare social worker. The primary focus would be the reliability of the narrative from the aunt of the 16-year-old boy. She should be able to provide information about the grounds for her suspicion. For example, can she describe occasions on which her suspicion was aroused and whether there was any disharmony between the sisters, what the sister's view was about the sexual relations in the family, the grounds for her suspicion about the sexual relationship between the father and his mother-in-law, and whether she herself had been sexually abused. It would be important to calm the situation as much as possible, inform the family that the case was being investigated, and reassure the sister that she had acted correctly by expressing her concern. It is also necessary to review the mental status and motives of the narrator.

The social worker would begin to chart the case immediately. A meeting would be arranged with her supervisor and colleagues, and the team would agree on how to continue. Collection of the background information about the situation of the family would be initiated. In Finland, the family has the right to be informed of the identity of the person reporting the account to the child welfare authorities. If it proves necessary to commence an investigation, the family would be met with, the situation assessed, and child welfare measures initiated. If the account of possible sexual abuse proved to be groundless—taking other reports into account—the child welfare services might send the family for therapy.

If there were reasons to suspect sexual abuse, depending on his physical and mental health and age, the social worker would arrange an interview with the 16-year-old boy. The focus would be on the protection and circumstances of the boy. If supporting evidence of sexual abuse was found, urgent child welfare measures would be taken, and the everyday life of the boy assured, for example, by placing him in a suitable family home or another place where he could continue his usual daily life. A criminal investigation would be requested from the police. In cases in which there is a strong suspicion of crime, it is important that the child be removed from the immediate environment of the suspect. The police would commence their own investigation process. If it proved necessary for the Child and Adolescent Psychiatry Forensic Unit to make an investigation, it would begin with a network meeting of the research group, the police, and the municipality's child welfare social worker. The duty of the latter would be to provide the preliminary information concerning the incident, as well as the history and living conditions of the family and the background information about the child.

In an examination of sexual abuse, the physician and psychologist would concentrate on the child. A somatic examination would be made and gynecological and surgical consultations would take place. The child's mental health would be examined by the psychiatrist from the Forensic Psychiatry Unit. The psychologist would assess the cognitive and personality development of the child and the social worker would talk with the adults involved in the case. She/he would also make an assessment of the family, which would include the family history, living conditions, and mutual interaction. In addition to the interview, the investigators would also use international assessment tools such as depression inventories for children and adults.

During the investigation process, the social worker would be in contact with the relevant professional network, in particular the child welfare social worker and counselors and teachers at school. Generally, a feedback meeting would take place with the child welfare officials of the municipality and the municipal social worker would carry out an assessment of the need for a child welfare intervention. A child welfare professional would continue working with the child and the family as necessitated by the investigation. Open care measures, such as economic support and care or therapy services, would be offered to the family. In the case of this 16-year-old boy, he would be supported towards independence by education, work, housing, and psychiatric care. If the mother were found guilty, the safety of the younger children would also be guaranteed. A social worker would work with the family, probably for many years.

Case study #3

Incest

BY KWAKU OSEI-HWEDIE AND MORENA J RANKOPO FROM BOTSWANA

Tebogo is a 15-year-old student who lives in a household with her grandfather, her mother, and her 12-year-old brother. Her father deserted them when she was five years old. For the past ten years, Tebogo's family has been living with her 65-year-old grandfather, Jakobe, who owns a bottle store and butchery in the village. He is well respected as a prominent community leader.

Tebogo is four months pregnant and went to a local social worker to help her obtain a legal abortion. She wants to continue with her education and does not want to be separated from her family. However, she does not want to reveal the man responsible for her pregnancy. She also does not want her mother or grandfather to know that she is pregnant. After extensive discussion with the social worker, she finally agrees that her mother must be informed and participate in the decision-making process about the pregnancy.

However, upon hearing that her daughter was pregnant, Tebogo's mother said that the social worker should leave them alone and that they would resolve the case within the family. The social worker insisted that, since the girl was a minor, this might be a case of incest or abuse which might require the involvement of the law. The mother then decided to cooperate with the social worker and convinced Tebogo to open up and talk freely so that they could get help. Subsequently, Tebogo explained that she was impregnated by

Jakobe, her grandfather. Upon hearing this, Tebogo's mother broke down. In between sobs, she told the social worker that Tebogo was the daughter of the grandfather, herself having been abused by her father.

Incest: A Social Worker from the US Responds

BY CHRISTIAN SARVER

Prevalence and Incidence

The prevalence of child sexual abuse in the US is difficult to pinpoint because of methodological issues in data collection (Administration for Children, Youth and Families [ACYF], 2007) and victims' reluctance to report, especially when the perpetrator is a family member (Mildred & Plummer, 2009). Research indicates that at least one in four girls and one in six boys will be the victims of sexual abuse before they turn 18 (National Center for Victims of Crime [NCVC], 2008), although that number includes all forms of sexual abuse. Cases where the perpetrator is a family member constitute one-third to one-half of sexual abuse against girls and one-fifth of abuse against boys (Finkelhor, 1994). In the US, cases of incest are investigated by child protective service agencies. Nationally, those agencies substantiated 905,000 cases of abuse by a caregiver in 2007, of which 8.8 per cent (approximately 79,640 incidents) were sexual abuse (ACYF, 2007). Of those cases, 27 per cent of the perpetrators were the child's parent and 29 per cent were a relative other than a parent.

Although children are most at risk for sexual victimization when they are between 7 and 13 years of age (Finkelhor, 1994), 40 per cent of sexual abuse cases that are substantiated by child protective services involve a victim between the ages of 12 and 17 (Wordes & Nunez, 2002). Low-income families have higher rates of child sexual abuse; although research suggests that such rates result from increased contact with social services by low-income families when they access public services (McDaniel, 2006).

Country Policies

Since the 1970s, federal law has shaped states' responses to child abuse, including sexual abuse. While states are given flexibility in handling incidents, the 1974 Child Abuse Prevention and Treatment Act (CAPTA) sets minimum standards for defining abuse and funds investigation, treatment, and prevention efforts. In order to receive federal funds, states must establish a system of mandated reporting, which means that certain professionals, including social workers, are required to report incidents of suspected child sexual abuse to designated authorities, most frequently law enforcement or child protective services (McDaniel, 2006). Mandated reporting laws supersede laws protecting client confidentiality and social workers risk civil or criminal charges for failing to make a report (Howing & Wodarski, 1992). Social workers might be involved in child sexual abuse cases in a variety of ways: they investigate claims as caseworkers with child protective services; they provide evaluation and support services as members of coordinated response teams; and they refer cases to the child welfare system in their work for agencies, schools, health care facilities, and in private practice.

Within child protective services, the social work response to incest is focused on assessing whether the child is at risk for continued abuse in the home. The 1997 Adoption and Safe Families Act, as well as CAPTA, dictate that child protective service social workers conduct their investigation in a manner that causes minimal disruption to the child, identify the family's strengths and supports the family's role in setting goals, and coordinate a range of support services (Golden, 2000). Federal guidelines, as well as standards set forth by the National Association of Social Workers (NASW), prioritize social workers' training in cultural competence, and require attention to cultural differences when assessing appropriate behavior and determining whether to remove a child from the home (NASW, 2008).

A Social Worker Responds

A social worker in this case must balance state and federal reporting requirements with agency policy and professional guidelines set forth by the social work code of ethics (NASW, 2008).

In most states, social workers are mandatory reporters and would be required to report suspected incest to child protective services or law enforcement agencies. While this reporting requirement supersedes Tebogo's expectation of confidentiality with the social worker, it could jeopardize the social workers' relationship with Tebogo and her mother.

To maintain a strong client relationship, a social worker might employ several strategies to empower the family throughout the reporting process, including: letting Tebogo and her mother know about the social worker's reporting requirements before abuse is disclosed; reminding them of reporting requirements once abuse is disclosed; inviting Tebogo's mother to report the abuse herself with the social worker's assistance; and giving accurate and comprehensive information about what will happen after the report is made.

Throughout this conversation, a social worker would offer validation and support to Tebogo and her mother.

Once the child discloses information that leads the social worker to suspect incest, she or he would report the incident to authorities, as designated by state law, and would not conduct any further investigation. While making the report, the social worker will be asked questions about the exact nature of the incident, the identity of the perpetrator, potential witnesses, and whether the abuse is ongoing; the social worker might also be expected to testify in court during civil or criminal proceedings. The social worker's employer might require him or her to consult with a supervisor before reporting the incident. Some agencies, primarily health care facilities, have in-house investigative teams that conduct interviews and medical evaluations; that team would then contact child protective services if it found evidence of abuse. While agency policy might require a social worker to consult a supervisor or an in-house department before making a report, state and federal law and social work licensing boards usually require that the social worker ensure that a report is made if he or she suspects abuse whether the supervisor concurs or not.

Once a report is made, it is the child protective service social worker's responsibility to conduct an investigation, during which Tebogo and her brother may be temporarily removed from the home, to determine how to keep the children safe from future abuse and if the grandfather will face charges. During this process, the original social worker's continued work with the family depends on the mission of the agency for which he/she works. The social worker might be contracted by child protective services to provide support to the family. Incest threatens an individual's emotional and social development, and the social worker would assess Tebogo to see how the incident has affected her social functioning, school performance, and mental health. The reporting process can also trigger guilt and anxiety for the survivor, who may feel responsible for getting the grandfather into trouble. Supportive interventions might include individual or family therapy for Tebogo and /or her mother. To enhance Tebogo's mother's ability to protect her children from future abuse, the social worker might provide services such as individual therapy, parent training, and peer support groups.

The social worker may also have an ongoing relationship with the family because she or he works in a school or community health center and thus would assess Tebogo and the rest of the family to determine the impact of both the abuse and the investigation by child protective services. Possible social work roles in this capacity include ensuring that Tebogo receive medical care for her pregnancy and working with Tebogo and her mother, so long as the mother is considered by the state to be a non-offending parent, to facilitate her decision-making process around the pregnancy.

The grandfather's removal from the home could threaten the family's economic well-being and the social worker would ensure that their basic needs—in terms of food, shelter, and transportation—are met. If Tebogo and her brother have been removed from the home, the social worker would facilitate the children's ability to maintain contact within important relationships, including friends, relatives, and their mother, so long as the mother is considered a non-offending parent.

Incest: A Social Worker from the Netherlands Responds

BY GUIDO VAN DE LUITGAARDEN

Prevalence and Incidence

The most recent prevalence study that could be found dates back to 1988 (Draijer, 1988) and indicates that 33 per cent of all girls have suffered some type of sexual abuse before the age of 16. Of all girls in the Dutch population, 15–16 per cent have been sexually abused by someone within the nuclear family, most often by a brother. Incidence figures could not be found. It should be stated that a rather broad definition of sexual abuse is used in this analysis, which means that sexual abuse is considered to include more than sexual intercourse alone, such as unwanted touching or kissing.

Country Policies

The Netherlands have a history of social work which dates back to the nineteenth century when social workers were first employed by the church and later by the state to combat poverty, resocialize criminals, and protect children. The status of a specific category of social workers, called "Maatschappelijk Werkers" (which could be translated as "societal workers") is recognized, whereas other groups of social workers do have their own academic education programs but do not have a legal status or a professional body to which they belong. The Netherlands has an elaborate and complex system of social services that can be provided in the case of intra-familial sexual abuse, including a child protection system, a variety of child welfare services, family services, mental health services, and perpetrator-focused interventions.

A Social Worker Responds

Assuming that the social worker mentioned in the case would be a "maatschappelijk werker," which is a type of generic social worker, he/she would first make an exploration of the situation. Subsequently, after consulting colleagues about this case, it is likely that a referral would be made to an Advies en Meldpunt Kindermishandeling (AMK), which provides advice and serves as a point of first referral in cases of suspected child abuse. Separate courses of action can be expected regarding each person involved, as each plays a different role in the case. In addition, family oriented interventions could be offered as a result of the impact that sexual abuse has on family relations. These initial steps in the case of suspected child abuse, neglect, or domestic violence are mandatory, since there is a law (Wet Meldcode Huiselijk Geweld en Kindermishandeling) that states that every organization in the fields of health and social care has to have a protocol that prescribes how these steps are to be taken within the specific context of the organization. These steps consist of: making an inventory of signals; consulting colleagues or the aforementioned AMK in order to eliminate that which is irrelevant to the case; and deciding to offer help or refer to the AMK.

To ensure the safety of the mother and her two children, as well as to initiate help, it would be possible to eject Jakobe from the family home for a maximum of ten days on the basis of a specific law (Wet op het Tijdelijk Huisverbod) which enables the mayor or, by delegation, an assistant district attorney to do this. This period of ten days can be extended to a maximum of four weeks if necessary. In addition, Jakobe could be arrested and prosecuted if he is charged with sexual abuse by the mother, Tebogo, or a social worker. In the case of child sexual abuse, the child welfare agency or the child protection board will report the alleged perpetrator to the police, unless this would conflict with the best interests of the children.

The position of the mother in this case would be particularly ambiguous as, on the one hand, she has been a victim of sexual abuse herself, but on the other could possibly be labeled as a neglectful mother for failing to protect her daughter. Depending on the extent of the psychological impact of the abuse she has suffered herself, she will be offered some form of mental health or counseling intervention to enable her to cope with her own traumatic past as well as her retraumatization as a result of discovering her daughter's victimization. In addition, being the adult responsible for the safety and well-being of her children, she will likely be assessed by child welfare workers as a first point of reference for child abuse (Advies en Meldpunt Kindermishandeling) with regard to her ability to protect her children against future abuse. If she is found to be a capable mother, a social worker from either the aforementioned agency or a women's refuge will talk with the mother about future living arrangements for herself and her children, as well as additional voluntary help in coping with the abuse and preventing it from happening again in the future. If the mother chooses to keep on living in the same house with her abusive father, and child welfare workers are not convinced that she will be able to keep her children safe in such a situation, forced help will be installed, and a family supervision order (Ondertoezichtstelling), possibly supplemented by an out-of-home placement (Uithuisplaatsing) for both Tebogo and her younger brother, is likely to be petitioned to a judge by the child protection board (Raad voor de Kinderbescherming). This action will be done at the request of the child welfare agency (Bureau Jeugdzorg) under which the aforementioned point of first referral resides. Before these measures are taken, an independent judge will have to consider the case, and decide on the request.

This process would also be the case if the mother is assessed as an inept mother by the child protection board. A family supervision order entails a limitation of parental custody over the involved children and important decisions about the children can only be made in cooperation with the responsible "family guardian" (gezinsvoogd). This guardian can also give the mother directives which she will have to obey. Family supervision orders are geared towards family intervention with the prospect of full custody being returned to the mother if the intervention is successful. If she refuses or is unable to cooperate, custody can be taken away from her and the children removed from the home. Although preference is usually given to voluntary acceptance of help by the family, if the parent is not willing or able to make use of such help, the aforementioned legal measures can be taken to impose assistance upon the family. If the mother chooses to live elsewhere with her children, initial shelter could be offered by a women's refuge. More structural solutions to this housing issue are subsequently dealt with by a social worker from the women's refuge or by a "maatschappelijk werker" who will try to make arrangements with a social housing cooperation.

The situation of Tebogo and her younger brother will be highly dependent on whether a family supervision order is given or even an out-of-home placement is imposed by a judge. If no such measure is taken, the children are likely to be offered one or more interventions by a child welfare agency or a psychologist if this is needed. If a family supervision order is given, the family guardian, together with the mother, Tebogo, and her brother, will discuss options for ensuring the safety of the children. The grandfather would be included in this process as well, if the mother would allow him to continue living with the family, although this is unlikely to be considered acceptable by the child welfare agency. If an out-of-home placement is ordered by a judge for one or both children, they would be placed in a children's home or in foster care. Considering the differences between the two siblings in this case, the fact that Tebogo is pregnant, and the difficulties in finding a foster family that would want to foster two teenagers, it would be highly likely that the children would be placed in separate foster families or homes.

Tebogo's situation has medical, psychological, and social aspects, of which the latter two would be addressed by social workers from a child protection or child welfare agency. She will most likely also be counseled regarding whether to have the baby. She will be informed in detail about the benefits and disadvantages of having an abortion, as she is 16 weeks pregnant and abortion is legal in the Netherlands until the twenty-fourth week of pregnancy. In practice physicians, will usually not perform an abortion after the twenty-second week of pregnancy. If she chooses to have the child, she will be able to either live with her family and have the baby looked after by them or a daycare center while she herself returns to school, as it is mandatory for children under the age of 16 to attend school. Special daycare arrangements are available for children of teenage mothers. If it is not possible for Tebogo to raise her child within her own environment or additional support is needed for Tebogo to fully assume her role as a mother, she could be placed in a residential group for teenage mothers and their children for a set period of time. This placement could start before childbirth and Tebogo would be guided during pregnancy, childbirth, and in raising her child. Medical and psychological attention would be given to the well-being of the newborn as well as the mother. Because Tebogo will be under the age of 18 when her child is born, the child protection board will provide a judgment with advice on who is to have custody of her baby. Depending on whether she is seen as a suitable mother by the child protection board, Tebogo's mother could be eligible to obtain custody of her daughter's child.

If the mother chooses to keep on living in the same house as her father and the children, and if this would be allowed by the child protection agency, a so-called CLAS (Contextual Learning groups for all those involved in cases of sexual abuse) intervention is likely to be initiated. This intervention aims to restore family relations while at the same time giving recognition to past injustices and wrongdoing within families where sexual abuse has occurred.

If Jakobe were to be legally prosecuted for sexual abuse, and if he were convicted, the judge might order a psychiatric evaluation of Jakobe to determine whether he can be held fully accountable for his actions. If he is shown to be psychiatrically ill, he could be sent for detention to a psychiatric hospital in addition to a prison sentence. After his release, he would be supervised by probation services.

Exercises

In class

The following topics for classroom discussion may be used bearing in mind that opinion and perspectives will differ. Exploration and discussion should be carried out in an atmosphere of respect and mutual tolerance in order to provide an effective forum for rewarding and fruitful debate.

- If you were the social worker involved in any one of these cases, how would you address related issues? Examine the similarities or differences in your response from those advanced by the case analysts.
- Explore the cultural and environmental differences between your community and those of the analysts and examine their relationship to the mode of intervention.
- What do you believe should be done to improve the response to the needs of children in your area of operation?

Out of class

For each of the exercises below select a country different from your home country and the countries discussed in this chapter. Present your findings to your peers in class on the following:

- Search for information about another country that provides insight into issues of child welfare and summarize the major current challenges to the society concerned.
- Consider the legal aspects of child welfare concerns in another country and compare them to those in your home country.
- Conduct a comparative literature review of two countries and their approach to matters surrounding child welfare and well-being, drawing conclusions of interest to social workers in those countries.
- Develop a list of agencies in your country that support children in need of care, identifying the gaps that require attention and making suggestions for addressing them.
- Obtain the views of two social workers in your community on issues of child vulnerability and identify significant aspects of the community's formal and informal response.

References

Child Rights Regulation 2002, Ghana.

Child Welfare Act 2007, Finland. No. 417.

Children's Act 1998, Ghana. No. 560.

Children's Act 2009, Botswana. No. 8.

Children in Need of Care Regulations (2005). Children's Act 1981 (Botswana).

Department of Social Welfare (DSW) (n.d.). Archives, Ashanti Region, Kumasi, Ghana.

Domestic Violence and Victims Support Unit (DOVVSU) of the Ghana Police Service, Sunyani Records (2010). Retrieved from http://www.ghanadistricts.com/news

Draijer, P. J. (1988). "Seksueel misbruik van meisjes door verwanten: Een landelijk onderzoek naar de omvang, de aard, de gezinsachtergronden, de emotionele betekenis en de psychsiche en psychosomatische gevolgen." [Sexual abuse of girls by relatives: A nationwide inquiry into the extent, nature, family backgrounds, emotional meaning and psychological and psychosomatic consequences.] Den Haag: Ministerie van Sociale Zaken en Werkgelegenheid, 587–88.

Early Childhood and Development Policy 2006. Ghana.

Ellonen, N., Kääriäinen, J., Salmi, V., & Sariola, H. (2008). "Violence against children and adolescents in Finland." Report No. 71. Publications of National Research Institute of Legal Policy and Police College of Finland.

Esping-Anderson, G. (2002). "Towards the good society, once again?" In G. Esping-Anderson, D. Gallie, A. Hemerijck, & J. Myles (Eds.). Why we need a new welfare state? (Oxford, UK: Oxford University Press), 1–25.

Finkelhor, D. (1994). "Current information on the scope and nature of child sexual abuse." The Future of Children, 4 (2), 31–53.

Gelles, R. J. (2007). "Introduction: Child abuse – an overview." In R. E. Clark, J. F. Clark, C. Adamec, and K. Mastel. (Eds). The encyclopedia of child abuse. (New York, NY: Facts on File Inc.)

Golden, O. (2000). "The federal response to child abuse and neglect." American Psychologist, 55 (9), 1050–53.

Government Bill for the Act on the organizing of the investigation of sexual crimes against children 2008, Finland No. 126.

Hélie, S., Clément, M.-E., and Larrivée, M. C. (2003). "Epidemiological considerations in the conceptualization and utilization of 'prevalence' and 'incidence rate' in family violence research: A reply to Brownridge and Halli (1999)," Journal of Family Violence, 18 (4), 219–25.

Helweg-Larsen, K. (2009). Framework for Nordic youth surveys on child sexual abuse and exposure to violence outside and in the family. (Copenhagen: Nordic Council of Ministers).

Hinkkanen, V. (2009). Sexual abuse of children: A study of sentencing practices and sexual reconvictions. National Research Institute of Legal Policy. Research Communications 92.

Howing, P. T., & Wodarski, J. S. (1992). "Legal requisites for social workers in child abuse and neglect situations." *Social Work*, 37 (4), 330–338.

Humppi, S.-M., & Ellonen, N. (2010). *Child abuse: The detection of cases, crime procedure and cooperation between authorities.* Tampere: Publications of Police College of Finland.

India Penal Code, Section 376 (1860). Retrieved from http://www.indian-kanoon.org/doc/1279834/

Information Technology Act, 2000 (India). Retrieved from http://unpan1.un.org/intradoc/groups/public/documents/apcity/unpan010239.pdf

Juvenile Justice (Care and Protection of Children) Act, 2000 (India). Retrieved from http://wcd.nic.in/childprot/jjact2000.pdf

Legal Aid Scheme Act 1997. Ghana. No. 542.

McDaniel, M. (2006). "In the eye of the beholder: The role of reporters in bringing families to the attention of child protective services." *Children and Youth Services Review*, 28 (12), 306–324.

Mildred, J., & Plummer, C. A. (2009). "Responding to child sexual abuse in the US and Kenya: Child protection and children's rights." *Child and Youth Services Review*, 31 (2), 601–8.

Ministry of the Interior (2008). "Safety first: Internal security programme." Publication 25, Finland.

Ministry of Women and Child Development (MWCD) (2007). "Child sexual abuse report." India. Retrieved from http://wcd.nic.in/childabuse.pdf

Mitta, M., & Singh, S. (2009). "India's gay day." Retrieved from http://epaper.timesofindia.com/Repository/ml.asp?Ref=Q0FQLzIwMDkvMDcvMDMjQXIwMDEwMA==&Mode=HTML&Locale=english-skin-custom

National Association of Social Workers (NASW) (1999). *Code of Ethics.* USA: NASW

National Association of Social Workers (NASW) (2008). USA: NASW. Retrieved from http://www.socialworkers.org/pubs/code/default.asp

National Center for Victims of Crime. (2008). "Child sexual abuse." Retrieved from http://www.ncvc.org/ncvc/main.aspx?dbName=DocumentViewer&DocumentID=32315

Niemi, H. (2007). "Sexual crimes against children and subteens." In National Research Institute of Legal Policy, No. 229. *Crime and criminal justice in Finland*, 85–93.

Niemi, H. (2010). "Sexual crimes against children and subteens." In National Research Institute of Legal Policy, No 250. *Crime and Criminal Justice in Finland*, 107–17.

Nursing Research Foundation (2008). *Recommendations for the Prevention of Interpersonal and Domestic Violence: Recognise, Protect, and Act.* Finland.

Ruiz-Casares, M., & Heymann, J. (2009). "Children home alone unsupervised: Modeling parental decisions and associated factors in Botswana, Mexico, and Vietnam." *Child Abuse and Neglect*, 33, 312–23.

United Nations Organization (1989). "Convention on the Rights of the Child." Author.

Wordes, M., & Nunez, M. (2002). "Our vulnerable teenagers: Their victimization, its consequences, and directions for prevention and intervention." Retrieved from http://www.nsvrc.org/es/publications/reports/our-vulnerable-teenagers-their-victimization-its-consequences-and-direcitons-pr

3 Couples Communication

By Joanna E. Bettmann

Communication is a hallmark of human development, because it is essential for survival and for creating and maintaining relationships among humans. However, patterns of communication vary along developmental and gender lines (Ashford & LeCroy, 2010) with positive interaction and communication patterns being key to productive dyadic relationships (Nelson, 2010). About 90 per cent of humans prefer to be married or partnered (United Nations, 2000), but these relationships can be problematic. Some of the issues that plague marriages and romantic relationships include conflict in communication and infidelity. In some instances, these issues stem from dysfunctional interactions, while in other instances dysfunctional interactions are only a consequence. Regardless of whether they constitute a consequence or causal factor of problems in relationships, dysfunctional interactions are often a reason for which people seek therapeutic support (Nelson, 2010). The resolution of marital conflict happens differently across cultures. In some places, couples seek the help of older family relatives or other elders, members of the clergy, or community leaders. This chapter focuses on couples communication and presents examples of ways in which social workers from different countries respond to some common issues in marriages or partnerships, including communication problems, infidelity, HIV infection, sexuality, and spirituality.

Communication Problems in a Couple

BY MIKA BARBER FROM THE US

Erik and Ashley have been married for two years. Erik is a 38-year-old school teacher. Ashley is 33 and is not working as she is pregnant with their first child. Ashley is excited about the upcoming birth and has been preparing by shopping and purchasing all the items they will need for their new baby. Prior to getting pregnant, Erik and Ashley spent much of their time traveling and pursuing mutual hobbies such as kayaking and windsurfing. Lately, Ashley is feeling frustrated with Erik's behavior. Erik has been spending more and more time at work and with his friends, and is rarely home. Ashley feels as though Erik is not available for her and is not part of planning for the baby. She has concluded that he must not be excited to have a baby. Ashley is feeling isolated and alone, and spends time each day crying in private. Erik's behavior is not only peculiar and out of character, but Ashley is worried that it will continue even after the baby is born. Erik is having some issues of his own with Ashley. He is feeling very stressed about the financial responsibilities that come with having a baby. He is worried that the small salary he earns as a teacher will not be enough to provide for his wife and new child. He feels frustrated that Ashley is spending too much money on baby items, some of which he believes are not needed. He is also feeling anxious about how the baby will change their ability to travel and pursue their hobbies as they have done in the past. Erik keeps all this to himself because he does not want to worry or stress Ashley. He knows that would not be good for her while she is pregnant. They decide to see a social worker about the issues between them.

Communication Problems in a Couple: A Social Worker from Indonesia Responds

BY CORNELIUS SISWA WIDYATMOKO & RETNANINGRUM RETNANINGTYAS FROM INDONESIA

Prevalence and Incidence

The authors were unable to locate any epidemiological studies about relationship problems in Indonesia. But based on a study on the psychological consultation rubric in one of the biggest national newspapers, data show that between 1998–2002, 17.71 per cent of readers' letters were complaints about relationships between husbands and wives (Eviandaru & Widyatmoko, 2004).

Country Policies

Indonesia is a developing country with a collectivistic culture. As a collectivistic society, the role of the extended family is important and is perceived as a potential resource. Thus people believe that children are not a burden for the family. One culturally-held notion is "banyak anak banyak rejeki," meaning "more children bring more fortunes." Another saying is "setiap anak membawa rejeki sendiri-sendiri," meaning "every child brings his/her own fortune." Indonesian people generally believe that children bring good things to families.

As a developing country, Indonesia is trying to improve its social services in health, education, and the economy. However, in comparison to services provided by private businesses, the government's public service is ineffective. Public services are slow, procedures unclear, and bribes to civil servants common, which creates a skeptical view of government services.

Social work in Indonesia is emerging as a profession. Most Indonesian people do not know what a social worker is or what help they could expect from such a professional. Currently, the Ministry of Social Affairs recruits and trains new social workers. Applicants have various undergraduate educational backgrounds including sociology, education, community development, and psychology. After acceptance into the Ministry of Social Affairs training program, they are briefly trained in social work, and then they work in local offices. Usually they work collaboratively with other social workers in a particular site, for example in shelters for natural disaster survivors to help them obtain sufficient aid. They also work in drug rehabilitation centers running programs for drug addicts and other inmates.

A Social Worker Responds

In the case of Ashley and Erik, the social worker needs to find a place for meeting with them because these workers do not have permanent private rooms to meet with clients. As soon as the social worker has gotten an appropriate place, he/she could start a counseling session.

A general counseling plan would be to first have individual sessions for Ashley and Erik, and then another with both of them. A good start could be counseling for Ashley, because her case appears to be much more complicated. She has the dual task of dealing with her own problems and taking care of the baby in her womb. The social worker needs to create a relaxed and receptive atmosphere in the session so that he/she could ask about Ashley's feelings at the present moment and encourage her to talk about them. The social worker would need to actively listen and respond to both the content and the nonverbal aspects of Ashley's story. This sort of atmosphere and the social worker's stance should be created consciously in all the sessions.

Ashley might need to talk about her loneliness because she feels that Erik is not available for her. The social worker needs to accept this feeling and have discussions about things that might reduce her loneliness. He/she could remind Ashley that Indonesian culture is a collective one, and that the extended family is a significant part of every family. For instance, if they feel happy that their daughter is having a baby, Ashley's parents will take part in preparing for the coming baby. So, the social worker could ask: Has Ashley tried to talk to them about this problem? Do Erik's parents know about her pregnancy? The social worker could explain that, by informing their parents about her pregnancy, she could share her feelings with them while signaling to them that they could help her take care of the baby.

The social worker could ask whether Ashley knows that the Indonesian government has a "Posyandu" service for pregnant mothers and mothers with a child who is less than five years of age in every village ("Posyandu" stands for "Pos Pelayanan Terpadu," which literally means integrated service post, which is an integrated health center). In this government service, nurses or midwives go with paramedics to villages to provide health care services. Through this government service, mothers can have medical staff check the condition of their pregnancy regularly and receive food supplements without any charge. Through this service, Ashley could meet other pregnant mothers and public health officers so that she might not feel so alone.

Another part of Ashley's feeling is her worry that Erik is not excited about having a new baby. The social worker could address Erik's behavior by exploring whether he thinks that he has to bear all the financial costs of the baby alone because he is "kepala rumah tangga," the head of the family. The social worker could explain that this thought comes from Indonesian

patriarchal culture, in which men and women have their own gender obligations. From that cultural perspective, both men and women feel burdened
and cannot share their obligations with each other. To solve this issue, the
social worker could discuss ways that Ashley could do more to help deal with
the family's financial burden.

In sessions with Erik, the social worker could adopt an approach similar to
that employed with Ashley, letting Erik express his feelings openly. Because
Indonesian men tend to have difficulty expressing their emotions, the social
worker could begin the conversation by asking about various emotions
that Erik might be experiencing. Is he stressed, upset, confused, anxious?
Regarding financial issues, the social worker could ask what Erik has done to
solve that problem. If Erik is a state teacher, has he reported his marriage to
the personnel bureau? If so, he is entitled to receive a wife allowance, which
is typically an additional 10 per cent of his salary if he works in a government
office or for a good private company. Does Erik know that the Indonesian
government has a program to help mothers in delivering babies so that they
can give birth at little expense? The social worker could educate Erik about
these programs and connect him to these government resources.

Erik complains that Ashley spends too much money on baby items. The
social worker could address this concern as a gender issue. In Indonesia,
each gender grows up with different values and behaviors. For example,
Indonesian men might not understand women's concerns regarding raising
babies. Similarly, men might not know what items are needed for babies. The
social worker could create some homework for Erik so that he can ask Ashley
about what her purchasing plans are for the baby, what she will buy, and why
she thinks she needs to buy such items. As this task might be misinterpreted
by Ashley as Erik not trusting her, the social worker needs to instruct Erik to
explain that these questions are homework for "gender understanding." The
point here is not to scrutinize Ashley's purchasing, but to help Erik understand Ashley's perspective. To enhance Erik's understanding of Ashley's
concerns, the social worker could encourage him to accompany his wife
when she goes to purchase items for their baby. This action might reduce
Erik's tendency to spend too much time in his office or with his friends.
The social worker might cite the old Indonesian expression "setiap anak
membawa rejeki sendiri-sendiri," which means "every child brings his/her
fortune." Indonesian ancestors raised their children with that belief and
thus, it is good not to worry too much about the financial burdens of raising
babies because they bring so much to families.

Regarding Erik's concern that the baby will affect their previous hobbies,
the social worker could bring this issue up as a shared responsibility between
husband and wife. As Erik shows more understanding of Ashley's concerns,
she may show more concern for his time and space. The social worker could

ask whether Erik would feel happy if he seeks his personal enjoyment alone and without his wife and baby. The social worker could encourage Erik and Ashley to plan instead pleasant activities for the whole family. Before Erik and Ashley had a baby, they could spend more time on their hobbies but when they have a child, it is necessary to have an activity that everyone can enjoy together. The social worker could encourage Erik to ask his and Ashley's parents how they managed their free time while raising babies.

After having separate sessions with Ashley and Erik, the social worker could arrange for an encounter involving both of them. In this session, the focus would be to reinforce a shared understanding between Ashley and Erik on how to cope with their problems, such as a willingness to carry financial burdens together, involving their parents in supporting them during pregnancy and the post-partum period, and other issues that might emerge. Another potential focus for the session would be to make a "to do list", which could include regular visits by Ashley to "Posyandu" (the government health service for pregnant mothers) or Erik accompanying Ashley to buy baby items.

In closing, the worker could express his/her appreciation that Ashley and Erik decided to consult a social worker about their issue. As a way to improve public understanding about professional social work, the social worker could explain that it is appropriate for people who have such problems to ask for help from these professionals, who are trained to assist in difficult circumstances. Because the profession is not well-known in Indonesia, Ashley and Erik might never seek help from a social worker, instead approaching religious authorities or clergy, friends, or family members. Resources such as these may be helpful but, from the perspectives of social and mental health services, they do not have the appropriate capability to address such problems. Perhaps Ashley and Erik might ask for help from a psychologist, but this professional's help will merely be with the mental health aspect of the problem. Psychologists do not have the capability to integrate their services with the social services that the government provides in the way that social workers do.

Communication Problems in a Couple: A Social Worker from the United Kingdom Responds

BY SURIYA NAYAK & GABRIELLE HESK

Prevalence and Incidence

Recent data released by the British Office for National Statistics (ONS) reveal an increase in divorce among British married couples. In 2010 data, indicated an increase of 4.9 per cent from 2009. In 2009, there were 113,949 divorces, and in 2010 this increased to 119,589 (ONS, 2010). Similarly, the number of dissolutions of civil partnerships continues to increase (Ross, Gask & Berrington, 2011).

Country Policies

A principle of UK social work is to look beneath the symptom or presenting issue to find out how the problem is symbolic of other unconscious complexities (Philips, 2007). If the space and place we occupy produces us (Probyn, 2003), a social work response is a product of the social, cultural, and historical space and place of the UK. Furthermore, the space and place that produce social work, the space and place of the relationship between the social worker and the couple, and the space and place experienced by Erik and Ashley as individuals constituting the couple are interlinked. The social worker could use Bronfenbrenner's (1979) ecological model as a framework to explore how the dyad functions as a system within a wider socio-economic system.

The issues presented in the case study raise questions about the threshold levels for intervention. Due to a UK professional social work culture oriented towards safeguarding those in crisis or in danger, the case of Erik and Ashley may not be assessed as urgent enough to warrant social work intervention. It is clear that this is short-sighted, undermines the role of the social worker, and needs to change. In the UK, a midwife or obstetrician may pick up on the levels of stress that Ashley is experiencing as a pregnant woman and assess the potential harm to her unborn child. The Edinburgh Postnatal Depression Scale (1987) is a useful framework to use alongside a holistic bio-psycho-social approach (Sudbery, 2010).

Recommendations from a number of inquiry reports (Laming, 2003) are instrumental in shaping a restructure of UK social work practice and education. The UK Social Work Reform Board and Social Work Task

Force have introduced the "Professional Capabilities Framework." A key shift is the reorientation of social work practice from a reactive crisis intervention approach to a preventive, strengths-based approach through the development of a meaningful social work structure-service user relationship to prevent a crisis (Munro, 2011). It is vital that a social work response to perceived risk is anti-oppressive and anti-discriminatory (Munro & Calder, 2005).

A Social Worker Responds

The social worker could focus on underlying issues of attachment, loss, transition, and communication (Sudbery 2010). Casement comments that, "for each person there are always two realities – external and internal. External reality is experienced in terms of the individual's internal reality, which in turn is shaped by past experience and a continuing tendency to see the present in terms of the past" (Casement, 1985, p. 2). A social worker in the UK could work with Erik and Ashley to understand how the external reality of the pregnancy, financial and practical pressures, the social constructions of parenting, and discourses about the family are experienced through the lens of Erik and Ashley's internal world. Thus, issues that are manifest in the present cannot be disconnected from the past. The social worker could explore how early attachment experiences including being parented has a direct impact on and can be triggered by becoming a parent. Erik and Ashley need to understand the link between attachment experiences and their internal working model because this provides: (a) an idea about other people and what can be expected from them; (b) an idea about self; and (c) an idea about how self and others relate (Beckett, 2002).

Using this approach, the social worker can achieve three goals. First, the social worker can enable Erik and Ashley to become aware of how their own experience of parenting shapes their response to becoming a parent. Second, the social worker can enable Erik and Ashley to explore how their attachment experiences shape intimate communication processes across the life course. Third, the social worker and the service user can look beyond the presenting issues.

Erik and Ashley are struggling with loss in relation to identity and role. A UK social work response may draw on Erikson's (1982, 1987, 1995) psychosocial model of the life course as a series of interdependent yet quite distinct stages and transitions. A social worker could explore how Erik and Ashley have negotiated previous life stages. Hopson's (1976) model of transition details a cycle from immobilization to integration. The cycle includes emotional reactions such as being overwhelmed, in despair, elated, feeling self-doubt, reflection, and searching for meaning as inevitable aspects of moving from one position to another. Hopson's model could offer the social worker a framework to enable communication between the couple. Erik and Ashley are in a period of transition from dyad to triad, from being two individuals in a couple to becoming parents, from having the freedom to travel, pursue hobbies such as "kayaking" and "windsurfing," to the responsibility of parenting. In the UK, the Kubler-Ross (1997) stage of grief model is influential. These stages include denial, anger, bargaining, depression, and finally acceptance. The social worker could enable Erik and Ashley to identify which stage they are negotiating and how.

A UK-based social worker could enable Erik and Ashley to understand the task of loss and transition as a process. Worden (1992) and Sudbery (2010) identify the following tasks in this process: facing reality, working through emotions, adjusting to changes in role, status and identity, and reinvesting in the future. The social worker may use concepts from Stroebe and Schut (1999), "loss orientation" and "restoration orientation," to enable the couple to understand and navigate the transition (p. 11). Repeated references to time in the narrative indicate that Ashley and Erik are struggling to reorientate to the multidimensional complexity of their new situation. For example, they refer to "not working since," "prior to getting pregnant," "much of their time traveling," "spending more and more time at work," "spends time each day crying," "worried that it will continue even after the baby is born," and "pursue their hobbies as they have in the past." Clearly, the couple is having difficulty making the transition from that which was prior to the pregnancy to the future prospect of being parents. A social worker could use the Holmes and Rahe Social Readjustment rating Scale (1967) to identify the levels of stress being experienced and then plan how to manage this.

Detailed analysis of the case study indicates that communication is a core issue, for example, "Erik is rarely home," "Ashley feels like Erik is not available to her," "Ashley is feeling isolated and alone," and "Erik has been keeping all this to himself." Wilson, Ruch, Lymbery, and Cooper (2008), identify two levels to effective communication. The first level includes "attentive and accurate listening to the content of the communication" (p. 297). The second level includes "being aware of and responding to what is being communicated, both verbally and non-verbally" (Wilson et al., 2008, p. 297).

A social worker in the UK might take one of several different theoretical approaches. From a humanistic person-centered approach (Rogers, 1951, 1961), the social worker might use the core conditions of unconditional positive regard, congruence, empathy, being nonjudgmental, and having respect in order to facilitate the sessions and develop an understanding of what level the couple is communicating on. Howe comments that, "[E]mpathy and mutual mind-mindedness is at the heart of both sound psychological development and social competence" (Howe, 2005, p. 20). There appears to be a lack of emotional attunement (Koprowska, 2005) between Erik and Ashley. From a psychoanalytic approach, the social worker would focus on unconscious communication in the relationship through transference, counter transference, projection, and projective identification (Sudbery, 2010). Thus the social worker could model a reflective process of understanding unconscious communications between the couple. Moon (2004) identifies an outcome of the reflective process as "the making of decisions/resolutions of uncertainty, the solving of problems, empowerment and emancipation" (p. 84). From a UK context, reflection is core to social work practice.

Case study #2

HIV Infection Among Partners

BY NTHABISENG NKWE FROM BOTSWANA

Mr and Mrs Smith have been married for a year. They met at church and courted for six months before they married. Mr Smith is 30 years old and a prominent lawyer at a successful law firm in a major city. Mrs Smith is 28 years old and a teacher at a junior secondary school. Before they married, the couple underwent premarital counseling offered by the church which did not include HIV counseling. After a year of blissful marriage, Mr Smith started suggesting to his wife that they have a child and that they should go for an HIV test together. Mrs Smith said she was not ready to have children and managed to put the subject aside for three months. After three months, Mr Smith broached the subject again. This time, he did not allow the matter to be ignored any further. A week following their discussion, the couple went to a local HIV counseling and testing facility where they were counseled and tested together. The HIV results for Mrs Smith were positive and those of her husband were negative. When they arrived home, a distraught Mr Smith asked how this could be possible. Mrs Smith began sobbing. She confessed to him that, before she became a born-again Christian and joined the church, she was in a relationship with another man and engaged in unprotected sex. Mr Smith, who had also been in sexual relationships before he became a Christian, confessed to Mrs Smith that he joined the church because he was trying to escape from a world that is full of sin and HIV. Mr Smith was overwhelmed. He had joined the church because he wanted to save himself from HIV infection and married a woman whom he thought was "pure." He could not understand how this had happened. Six months after the HIV test, Mr and Mrs Smith have not resumed any sexual activity. Mr Smith says he is very confused since he feels that he has been betrayed by his church and by God. He says he does not want a divorce, but does not know what to do since he wants children and does not want to become infected. He says he still loves his wife very much. Mrs Smith is consumed by guilt and grief at the thought of the suffering she is causing her husband. There is now lack of trust in the relationship although they still have deep feelings for each other. The couple decides to speak with a social worker recommended by the HIV testing facility.

HIV Infection Among Partners: A Social Worker from the United Kingdom Responds

BY JILLIAN MURPHY

Prevalence and Incidence

In the UK, the number of people with HIV diagnoses as of June 2011 was 118,251 (Health Protection Agency (HPA), Health Protection Scotland, UCL Institute of Child Health, 2011). At the end of 2010, the estimated figure for people with HIV diagnoses in the UK was 91,500. Heterosexuals constituted 50 per cent of new HIV cases for this period with men who have sex with men (MSM) making up 45 per cent of the figure (HPA, 2011).

Country Policies

The UK's General Social Care Council regulates the social work profession, manages mandatory registration and enforces codes of practice. Social workers promote the full involvement and participation of service users to empower them in all aspects of decision making and action that affect them. Social workers in the UK aim to recognize the whole person, within family, community, and societal environments, and to empower people through the development of their strengths. Social workers in the UK also aim to promote social justice by challenging discrimination, recognizing diversity, challenging unjust policies and conditions that contribute to social exclusion, and working towards an inclusive society.

Social work is a profession that is not well understood by the British public. The British Equality Act of 2010 places a duty on social work to promote equality of opportunity for people living with HIV. Discrimination includes failure to make reasonable adjustments to enable the use of a service of the same quality and on the same terms as others. Those who "appear to be in need of community care services" are entitled to an assessment of need and the provision of care (NHS and Community Care Act 1990, S. 47 (1)). Disability in the UK is defined as a physical or mental impairment which has a substantial and long-term adverse effect on one's ability to perform daily activities. The British Human Rights Act of 1998 places obligations on social work to respect private and family life. The White Paper *Improving the life chances of disabled people* (Prime Minister's Strategy Unit, 2005) identifies appropriate service responses for families affected by HIV/AIDS (Department of Health, 2005).

Barriers of poverty, stigma, and poor information distribution prevent access to services for people living with HIV. People with HIV are twice as likely as others to live in low income households (Palmer, Carr & Kenway, 2005). Positive HIV status correlates with unemployment, difficulty accessing housing, and being refused a mortgage following diagnosis (Parker & Aggleton, 2002). Stigma against HIV, whether actual or perceived, can create reluctance in patients to seek support. Retaining control of their personal information is, therefore, a matter of acute concern to HIV patients (Anderson & Doyal, 2004). They will not always want confidential health information to be shared with others (Anderson, 2004).

A Social Worker Responds

Social work intervention would be offered within a framework of anti-discriminatory practice which is supportive, respectful and considerate. Intervention from a social worker should be easy to access, not stigmatizing, and should enhance informal support networks (Gardner, 2002). The social worker should consider conducting the assessment at the clients' home and incorporate a social model of disability that would address disabling barriers, and provide a range of interventions from which the couple could select to suit their needs.

Interventions would flow from an initial diagnostic and functional assessment which would determine the intensity of the intervention (group work, individual program, or combinations thereof). In order to ensure health, education, and social care it is essential that professionals communicate and work collaboratively to maximize effectiveness. Social work support would help the couple to focus on what is working, identify their hopes and goals for the future and facilitate a series of structured and monitored steps to achieve their goals. The social worker should focus on the clients' strengths and aspirations, as well as their difficulties. Clients may immediately need information, advice and advocacy regarding housing, benefits, and debt. The social worker could offer support relating to immigration status, finding a doctor, other health services such as counseling, and liaison with other agencies (Huntingdonshire Primary Care Trust, 2005).

The social work intervention with the Smiths could include a range of interventions. Counseling may cover HIV and AIDS information, the testing process, risk-reduction strategies, partner communication, and disclosure. One in five people in the UK have received such counseling and 65 per cent said it helped (National Survey of Sexual Attitudes and Lifestyles, 2001). Social work intervention might also include providing jargon-free information about health and how service providers can help. Intervention might also include acknowledging clients' reluctance to approach statutory agencies for help and encouraging them to consider support from non-governmental organizations. Intervention could also involve providing information about how services should be coordinated, information on advocacy services, advice on obtaining welfare benefits, or information on informal community networks. Intervention may involve couples counseling, group counseling for family members and peers, or referral to a self-advocacy or peer support group for individuals in similar positions. Intervention might also include encouraging the involvement of extended family members who might offer support.

People living with HIV have significant emotional needs and require support in coming to terms with their infection. Shock, anger, fear over disease progression and isolation by family and friends, and worries about infecting others would be expected by the Smiths. Depression is twice as common in people with HIV compared to the general population (Cook et al, 2004; American Psychiatric Association, 2008). Addressing the couple's emotional needs would facilitate positive outcomes, which can improve overall health, strengthen preventive behavior, and improve life chances. Finding ways to reduce symptoms of depression could potentially prolong and improve the life of the wife (World Health Organization, 2003).

Social work intervention with the Smiths would address coping with illness, communicating about the disease, strengthening conflict resolution skills, and planning for the future. The Smiths may worry about how their lifestyles will change and if it will be possible to have children. Counseling provided by a social worker would support their acceptance of the diagnosis and facilitate more effective absorption of information regarding disease consequences, leading to better-considered decisions about the future and treatment.

Individuals and caregivers who are well informed about HIV and the associated medical implications manage their illness better, and have an increasing ability to plan for the future (Horberg et al., 2007). Social work intervention with the Smiths should support disclosure to family, friends, colleagues, and health workers. The Smiths may be anxious about how others will react. They may also be concerned with avoiding discrimination, which creates little incentive to disclose. Disclosure planning with the social worker might include seeking advice from other HIV-positive people who have disclosed their status.

The social worker may also help the Smiths to prepare for treatment. People may live with HIV for many years after diagnosis with little or no noticeable change in their health. Eventually, however, it will be necessary to begin antiretroviral treatment which can be challenging considering that antiretroviral drugs will have to be taken daily for life. Treatment requires high degrees of commitment and means that the couple should be in a fit mental state before commencement (St. George's Pediatric HIV Team, 2003). Adjusting to a new treatment regimen which includes remembering dosage, frequency, and time of administration can be emotionally draining.

The social worker should also support the Smiths in family planning. From the start of the HIV epidemic through to June 2010, there have been 11,429 children in the UK born to HIV positive mothers. Of these children, only eight per cent have become infected with HIV (HPA, 2010). Early intervention, prenatal screening, treatment to block transmission, avoiding breastfeeding, and elective caesarean delivery all dramatically reduce the number of new cases. However, the social worker should address the Smiths' possible emotional burden of the fear of transmission.

The husband in this case is likely to experience emotional pain, grief, and concern about how the disease could affect his wife and their relationship, concern about how he can best support her and guilt for his own feelings. He would need specific support to come to terms with the diagnosis (*National Institute of Allergy and Infectious Diseases*, 2006). Discussing feelings with others including friends, church members, family, and support groups, learning about HIV, staying healthy, and making space and time to relax and take part in other activities can help. He may also have symptoms of anger and grief (Cairns, 2008). He might utilize avoidant coping strategies of substance abuse, denial, and withdrawal.

Social work intervention with Mr Smith would promote adaptive coping strategies such as finding support, developing communication, and finding meaning (WHO Media Center, 2006). Enabling the couple to grieve or mourn for as long as they need to would be managed to ensure that they are not overwhelmed by their situation. Caring for a person with HIV without adequate support places huge demands on the caregiver, with the possibility of it affecting his or her mental and social health and often resulting in mental and physical collapse. The husband would need support to manage the emotional burden associated with his dual role. Support groups and helplines would be able to offer help in allaying any anxieties that have resulted from rumors or misinformation and advice on all aspects of coping with HIV. Peer-support groups run by people with HIV enable those living with the virus to realize that they are not alone in what they are going through. These peer-support groups may be able to offer the best assistance.

HIV Infection Among Partners: A Social Worker from India Responds

BY ANISH K. R.

Prevalence and Incidence

India has a population of one billion, around half of whom are adults in the sexually active age group. The first AIDS case in India was detected in 1986 and HIV infection has since been reported in all Indian states and territories.

The National AIDS Control Organization releases HIV figures every year based on data gathered from HIV Sentinel Surveillance sites. In 2007, surveillance was conducted at 1,134 sites and 358,797 samples were tested for HIV. The estimates suggest national adult HIV prevalence in India is approximately 0.36 per cent, constituting between 2 and 3.1 million people. Higher percentages are found among people attending STD clinics (3.6 per cent), female sex workers (5.1 per cent), injecting drug users (7.2 per cent), and men who have sex with men (7.4 per cent). (NACO, 2008) The epidemic in India shows a declining trend overall. HIV prevalence among the adult population in 2007 was 0.34 per cent and in 2008 was 0.29 per cent (UNGASS, 2010).

Country Policies

The National AIDS Control Programme (NACP) is anchored in the National AIDS Prevention and Control Policy of 2002. The current NACP, Phase III which began in 2007 has well-articulated national strategies and approaches towards prevention, care, support, and treatment. The main goal of NACP was to halt and reverse the HIV epidemic in the country within a five-year period. The formulation of NACP Phase IV is in progress.

The NACP has decentralized the responsibilities for prevention, support, and supervision to the state, district, and sub-district levels, to ensure access to services across the country. The National AIDS Control Organization works closely with State AIDS Control Societies set up in each state to implement its mandate. District AIDS Prevention and Control Units are set up in some of the most vulnerable districts to provide management oversight to HIV and AIDS activities in the districts. Convergence of the NACP III with the National Rural Health Mission has been aimed at six areas, namely Integrated Counseling and Testing Centers; Prevention of Parent-to-Child Transmission; Blood Safety; Services for Sexually Transmitted Infections; Condom Programming; and Anti-retroviral Treatment (UNGASS, 2010).

The NACP Phase III used approximately US $2.5 billion from the contributions of World Bank, the UK Department for International Development, and the Global Fund against AIDS, TB and Malaria. It also pooled funds from the Government of India and private initiatives like the Bill and Melinda Gates Foundation. The NACO established Community Care Centres (CCC) for providing comprehensive care, support, and treatment services.

Professional social work practice in India started with the commencement of the social work program at the Sri Dorabji Tata Graduate School of Social Work currently known as Tata Institute of Social Sciences, in Mumbai in 1936. However, the Servants of India Society founded by Gopala Krishna Gokhale in 1905 is considered as the first major organization in the field of social work. The organization insisted on a scholarly study of the social problems for which they sought solutions. This development was a pioneering initiative for a rational and scientific approach to the solution of social problems (Gore, 1965; Desai, 2006). The ideologies of Indian professional social work have developed as a combination of modern professional values, Indian religious values, and ideologies, and values of the Gandhian Sarvoday movement (Desai, 2006).

Social work professional activities in India are developmental and clinical in nature. The developmental social work paradigm uses a macro-practice perspective which focuses primarily on poverty alleviation and helping to link people to resources with the aim of strengthening communities. Social workers maintain a special focus on empowering vulnerable groups like women, children, and the differently abled.

Indian clinical social work practices focus on mental health, health care, and industrial and HIV/AIDS scenarios. The clinical social work activities include individual counseling, family counseling, addiction counseling, psychotherapeutic interventions, and enhancing the linkage between resources and people. Mental health social workers focus on promotion of mental health, child guidance and counseling, school social work, rehabilitation, and clinical services for adults, children and families. Social work practice in health care is concentrated on palliative care and clinical services in all medical specialties.

A large number of social workers offer clinical services in HIV and AIDS prevention projects, HIV testing centers and HIV care, and support and treatment services. The National AIDS Control Organization has an array of services for the HIV infected and affected. Care and support for people living with HIV and AIDS is provided through Anti-retroviral Therapy Centers, Drop in Centers, Prevention of Parent- to- Child Transmission Counseling Centers, and Community Care Centers. Anti-retroviral Therapy Centers provide care and free drug treatment to HIV positive individuals, as well as counseling, nutrition support to women and children living with HIV, and social support. The National AIDS Control Programme funds these programs and services are free to recipients. The prevention programs mainly target individuals at risk for transmitting HIV, especially female sex workers, men having sex with men, and intravenous drug users. The care and support programs are offered to individuals who are identified with HIV infection and the antiretroviral treatment is offered to persons with HIV infection who have a CD4 count of 250 and below (NACO, 2010).

Community Care Centers play a critical role in providing treatment, care and support to people living with HIV and AIDS. Under National AIDS Control Programme Phase III, these centers are attached to Anti-retroviral Therapy centers and ensure that persons living with HIV and AIDS are provided: (a) counseling for ARV drug adherence, nutrition, and prevention, (b) treatment for opportunistic infections, (c) referral and outreach services for follow up purposes, and (d) social support services. The centers seek better community and family responses towards persons living with HIV and AIDS through family counseling. For better treatment outcomes, the centers provide families with counseling on patients' nutritional needs, treatment adherence, and psychological support.

A Social Worker Responds

The social worker would meet the clients in the community care centers, which is the primary contact place for the social worker and persons living with HIV in India. A social worker in India would initiate the session by building an alliance with Mr and Mrs Smith. The social worker would verbally appreciate the couple for making a joint decision to meet a social worker, explaining that this is a positive step towards resolving issues between the couple. The initial relationship-building phase of treatment would be followed by an assessment of the emotional status of Mr and Mrs Smith. The social worker would deal first with emotional aspects of the case in order to help the clients to make appropriate decisions and life choices.

The assessment is usually performed through observation and evaluation of the client's emotional status. Social workers also use standardized checklists or tools for identifying depression and anxiety among the clients. The social worker would empathize with Mr Smith regarding his wish to escape from the world of sin and HIV and the reality of having an HIV infected partner. Mr Smith's dilemma about his need for having a child and keeping him free from an HIV infection would be a focus of attention for the social worker. The social worker would note the couple's love for each other and willingness to continue in the relationship. The social worker's assessment would explore strengths of the marital dyad and support that is available from significant others and their social networks. This is because Indian social workers recognize the importance of clients' kin networks, since most often family ties are strong even after developing a family system of one's own. The social worker could also use support systems from the extended family in the process of helping. Hence the assessment includes the psychological functioning of the clients (intrapersonal), their family system, and the ecological systems.

The social worker would summarize the concerns shared by the couple, negotiate goals for the intervention. and enter into a contract with the couple. The contract is often informal and not written. The intervention with the couple would then focus on the resolution of the emotional issues and dilemmas of Mr and Mrs Smith. The social worker would create an environment of acceptance through attentive listening and reflection of feelings along with empathic responses. He/she would expect that the couple could overcome the current emotional issues through a supportive therapeutic environment. Social workers also employ methods of grief counseling/grief work to deal with emotional issues of persons living with HIV. After addressing the stress, depression, and anxiety associated with the present situation, the social worker would focus on building trust between the couple. A family strengths approach from a systemic perspective would be used in this context (Stinnett & DeFrain, 1985; DeFrain, 1999). The social worker would facilitate two to three couple sessions to help them to ventilate their feelings and emotions, which would help in reducing their distress.

In subsequent sessions, the social worker would reinforce the fact that both Mr and Mrs Smith do not want a divorce. The worker would motivate both of them to express how they care for each other and help the couple to conceptualize their concerns and needs. The social worker would further explore whether they could forgive each other for what had happened in the past, as well as assessing their readiness to work together to move forward in life. Perhaps, in this case, since both are Christians, the social worker could also utilize their belief system for the sake of intervention. The Christian belief of considering marriage as a covenant and a sacred relationship would be explored.

The social worker would also explore the issue of the husband wanting a child and discuss options for the couple to have a child without Mr Smith becoming infected. One option which the social worker would explore is referring the couple to a legal practitioner and an adoption agency for considering the possibility of adopting a child. This option would be difficult since adoption agencies may not approve adoption by an HIV-infected parent. Another option would be referring the couple to a doctor to explore the possibility of having a test-tube baby. A third option would be exploring with the couple whether the wife would be willing to have her husband's child through a donor mother. Finally, a fourth option would be exploring with the couple the possibility of artificial, intra-cervical, or intra-uterine insemination.

The social worker would refer the case to an Anti-retroviral Therapy Center for further treatment and support. The couple would also be referred to a community care center for pregnancy and child birth related issues. Ideally, the social worker would hold four to six sessions for resolving the emotional issues and facilitating decision making along the lines discussed above. The social worker would then terminate the case keeping options open for follow-up meetings as needed.

Case study #3

Spirituality in Partnership

BY KWAKU OSEI-HWEDIE & MORENA J. RANKOPO FROM BOTSWANA

Ben is a 27-year-old teacher who is accused by his girlfriend of abandoning her. Ben and Bonolo, a 22-year-old woman, have been dating for three years. But recently Ben has been spending increasing amounts of time with Marang, who is 35 and lives in the neighborhood. Marang works as a cleaner in their area. Bonolo believes that because she is more educated than Marang, as well as more beautiful, younger, dynamic, and a secretary, Ben should not leave her for Marang without a good reason. In the three years they have been together,

Bonolo has supported Ben and helped him financially and emotionally. She believes that she has made him the handsome young man that he is now. Bonolo has reported the matter to Ben's elder sister, Mary. Bonolo told Mary that she consulted a spiritual leader who revealed to her that Ben was bewitched by Marang, who had administered love potions to Ben through food. Bonolo also told Mary that Marang has been overheard boasting that no one can take Ben away from her because she is powerful, and that she does not mind eliminating her opponents through witchcraft. Bonolo wants Mary to intervene since she cannot directly approach Ben's parents. Mary agrees and approaches her parents to urge them to go to a traditional healer to ascertain the truth. Ben's parents finally agree as they are convinced that a man cannot have a love affair with an older woman without him being bewitched. However, Ben's aunt, a graduate and a civil servant, does not agree with the parents and maintains that Ben might have found his true love. In all this, Ben seems unconcerned and unbothered by what is happening around him. The parents then consult a spiritual healer who asserts that Ben and Bonolo are genuinely in love and that Ben must be assisted to come to his senses. At this point, Bonolo asks a social worker in her neighborhood to help Ben to do so.

Spirituality in Partnership: A Social Worker from Israel Responds

BY NEHAMI BAUM

Prevalence and Incidence

No figures of the prevalence or incidence of the type of problem described are available in Israel. The Department of Welfare policy is to respect the privacy of clients seeing social workers employed in the government sector. Similarly, the Code of Professional Ethics of Social Workers in Israel (2007) prohibits divulging information without the client's permission, except where there is danger to life or safety. Personally, I myself have never encountered any clients who spoke of witchcraft nor have any of my social work students had any such client in their fieldwork.

Country Policies

Israel is a multicultural society, where native Israelis mingle with immigrants from virtually every continent. The population is fairly evenly divided between persons of Western and Eastern cultural backgrounds with many variations of each. About 80 per cent of the population is Jewish and 20 per cent Muslim. For the most part, Israel is a technologically advanced, liberal Western democracy. Most of the Jewish populations are secular but Jewish history and values are integral to the country. Thus, the religiously-observant minority has considerable political power and a strong impact on daily life through the authority exercised by religious institutions over marriage, divorce, and the maintenance of Sabbath restrictions.

Israel has about a dozen schools of social work. In general, social work education follows the US model with a strong focus on clinical work. Because of the many different cultural groups that make up Israel's population, a great deal of emphasis is placed on teaching cultural sensitivity and cultural competence. A license as a social worker can be obtained upon the completion of an accredited three-year MSW program and is required for employment as a social worker. Although status as reflected in salaries and working conditions are not high, social workers regard and conduct themselves as serious professionals.

Social workers are employed in both the public and private sectors. Free psychological counseling for children and adults, as well as couple and family therapy, is provided through the municipal welfare departments in every city and town. The services are available to all who apply and no referral is necessary. Most clients using the public services are of low or middle socio-economic strata. Persons in the middle and upper socio-economic echelons tend to use services at private agencies.

A Social Worker Responds

In Israel, Bonolo is unlikely to have sought help with her problem from a social worker or any mental health professional. More likely, she would have sought out a religious figure or a self-styled healer, medium, or other person who claimed to have magical or spiritual powers. Moreover, if she did seek help from a public service, her application is likely to receive low priority in view of the fact that neither she nor anyone else involved in her unhappiness was at risk of physical or emotional harm, and she would have had to wait as much as a year to see a counselor.

If Bonolo did reach a social worker, the case would probably be handled in much the same way in both the public and private sector. In both settings, the social worker's first step would be to conduct a detailed intake procedure to hear how Bonolo defined the problem and to obtain preliminary information about her and the relationship. On the basis of this, he/she would then make her own psycho-social assessment. Whatever the evaluation, the social worker would certainly make it clear that under no circumstances would he/she initiate contact with Ben, his family members, or his friends. Unless the client was a minor, he/she would regard making unsolicited contact with other persons as both unhelpful and unethical.

The social worker would probably offer to meet with Bonolo to discuss her relationship with Ben and her feelings about having been left by him. Although she would not say so outright, it is unlikely that she would accept Bonolo's explanation that Ben left her because he was bewitched. She would view this explanation as an expression of Bonolo's feelings of loss of control and would direct the intervention towards helping her to regain a sense of control over her life.

In effect, to the extent that Bonolo allowed, the social worker would undertake therapeutic intervention. He/she would probably begin by encouraging Bonolo to ventilate so as to alleviate her anxiety and, at the same time, try to win her trust and form a therapeutic alliance with her. To enable such an alliance to develop, the social worker would first contain the anger and frustration that Bonolo would probably feel in the wake of her refusal to provide the type of assistance she had expected. Specifically, he/she would make space for Bonolo to express her feelings, listen empathically to them, and help her to bear their weight.

If he/she succeeds in creating a therapeutic alliance and Bonolo does not leave the therapy, the social worker would encourage Bonolo to explore her assumptions about the break-up of the relationship. Specifically, she would encourage Bonolo to examine her assumption that, after she had supported Ben emotionally and financially for three years, he had not left her of his own accord for a woman who was older, less educated and less pretty than she. The aim of this probing would be to help Bonolo regain her lost sense of control by helping her to understand her own contribution to the breakup. The hope would be that Bonolo would come to realize that her conviction that she "had made him the handsome young man that he is" is belittling and emasculating and may well result in her man feeling of little worth and potency. If Bonolo can realize this and change her behavior, she will be in a better position to form new and sounder relationships.

In the course of this exploration, the question of why Bonolo chose a partner who required or accepted her emotional and financial support would probably arise. What did she gain from being the giving person in the relationship? What did her choice of an emotionally and financially dependent man say about her own sense of self-worth? Moreover, at the intake, the social worker would probably have noted to herself the difference in the origin and affiliation of Bonolo's and Ben's names. In Israel, names often indicate their bearers' cultural backgrounds. The fact that the parties in an intimate relationship have names of different origins and affiliations may be significant. It may be a matter of chance and meaningless. It may reflect deep differences in the partners' culture and social status. If, in the course of the intervention, it turns out that the difference has meaning for Bonolo, the social worker might explore with her its role in her choice of Ben as her partner.

As apparent from the above account, the intervention would focus on Bonolo. It is likely that Bonolo would at times talk about Ben's behaviors and motives. The social worker would acknowledge and help to clarify Ben's role in the dynamic; however, he/she would maintain focus on Bonolo's motives and behavior.

Bonolo might continue to try to win Ben back or abandon her efforts to do so. She might or might not try to form another relationship. The social worker would not try to influence her decision. The social worker's hope would be that, whatever Bonolo decides to do, she now understands that she is not a helpless pawn and that things do not just happen out of nowhere, but that her own choices and behaviors play an important role in the shape her life takes. If the intervention continues beyond this point, the social worker's aim would be to help Bonolo to do the inner work necessary to form and maintain the type of relationship she wants. That is, together with Bonolo, he/she would explore what Bonolo needed and wanted in a close relationship, including needs and desires she may not have acknowledged even to herself. The social worker would hope that such understanding might enable Bonolo to choose a suitable partner for herself.

Spirituality in Partnership: A Social Worker from India Responds

BY KATY GANDEVIA & NAINA ATHALE

Prevalence and Incidence

For a large number of people in India, there is intrinsic faith in the supernatural as well as a strong belief in the afterlife, ghosts, and spirits. In many parts of the country, sorcery and faith healing is an important part of community life. The sorcerer and healer are consulted for many illnesses, or bad and tragic occurrences in families, and many practices like animal sacrifice. Many people use a talisman like a stone, a gem, a powder, or a potion as a penance or for curing illness. In some communities, there is also belief in black magic by witches. Women are often blamed for bad occurrences in families and villages and are then physically and mentally abused, sometimes leading to death. Many people have great faith in palmistry, astrology, and horoscopes. In fact, most of the important events in life are planned or kept track of with the help of astrologers. For example, astrologers help families plan arranged marriages, matching the horoscopes of both for compatibility before the marriage is finalized.

Some examples are more common in some religions and within certain castes and communities than others. However, it seems that overall no Indian religion or community is free from such beliefs or practices.

Country Policies

Since all of the beliefs and practices have their basis in old community cultures as well as in the practices of religion, India has not touched this area of civil life with any laws. Some practices are considered illegal under certain sections of the Indian Penal Code, if they are harmful or infringe on the rights of an individual. For example, the practices related to exorcizing of spirits from a person or tormenting a person for being a witch is illegal. Some states in the country have now drafted their own version of the Prevention of Blind Faith and Harmful Practices Act; the Central government is also in the process of drafting the same. However, it is important to note that many mental health practitioners believe that indigenous practices can be included in modern mental health interventions, provided they are accessed only for their helpful, not harmful, effects.

Indian civilization has been in existence for approximately 6,000 years. Socially and culturally, it is highly diverse. Hence, it is impossible to speak of a single, integrated Indian social structure. After Indian independence from Britain in 1947, the country saw momentous changes but in this environment, certain social realities remain. The first is the caste system. Several centuries ago, the caste system began as a grouping of people according to their occupations, which over time got labeled as "pure" (teaching, priesthood, ruling class, and business which formed the three upper classes) and the "non-polluting" but lower occupations like carpentry, weaving, and gardening. The "polluting" occupations like cleaning streets and toilets, collecting garbage, disposing of animal carcasses, or skinning animals were occupations that were out of the class system altogether, later known as the "outcastes." These classes which initially allowed some amount of movement between occupations later became rigid and turned into a tyrannical caste system, with no vertical mobility, involving victimization of the lower castes and the outcastes.

Marriages between castes were forbidden, and even now, a large part of the population does not approve of marriages outside one's own caste. Though the origins of the caste system are in Hinduism, this system has been adopted in most religions and communities in India. With its vertical form of rigid social stratification, it constitutes the basic feature of Indian society today. Inter-caste marriages are frowned upon. In more traditional parts of the country, such couples and their families are not allowed to participate in the social life of the community, leading to social isolation for the entire family.

In post-independence India, and with the formation of constitutional democracy, India has experienced a gradual change in societal attitudes. For example, the government opened the education system to all and barred discrimination in job hiring. These initiatives have gone a long way in freeing the tight restrictions of social movement in society. Yet, it is important to note that some occupations are still exclusively practiced only by certain castes, the so-called "polluting" ones.

A second important feature of Indian society is the well-entrenched social class which is strong even within the castes. India has a small elite upper class, which is rich, influential, and powerful. The country also has an increasingly large middle class which consists of educated professionals, government employees, and small or medium-sized business owners. In India, the largest class is the poorest: often powerless daily-wage laborers, people in small insecure contract positions, or landless laborers in rural areas working on the lands belonging to the upper castes. Unlike the caste system, movement within social classes is comparatively easy. This movement is possible when individuals gain financial independence and become successful in their professions.

A third important feature of Indian society is the family. The Indian family is generally large and extended. However, its structure and functions have undergone some changes, particularly in urban areas where the nuclear family has emerged with greater importance. In most Indian families, the extended family plays a critical role. For example, though they may live in separate homes with their families, brothers will make important joint decisions about family marriages and property. Further, the opinion of their extended family, community, and caste group will be of great importance in decision-making. In the Indian context, the emphasis during childhood socialization is on interdependence rather than independence, and this includes marriages. In all religions and communities, most marriages are arranged by the parents of the bride and the groom who act in consultation with the family and community elders. There are certain common practices cutting across religious and caste lines when it comes to these marriages. For example, the groom is almost always older and taller than the bride. The groom is also expected to earn more than the bride in case she is also an educated working woman. Additionally, horoscopes also have to be matched for compatibility before finalizing the marriage in almost all Hindu communities. There are changes now, especially in the urban areas and metropolises. But for a large part of the country, a marriage is still arranged within one's community with the approval of community elders.

Social work is a comparatively young profession in India even though social welfare historically has been an integral part of the Indian culture. Almost all the religions of the world originated on the Asian continent, and all of them advocated charity and compassion for the disadvantaged and the less fortunate in society. Thus, a welfare approach existed for centuries in India. In 1905, the Servants of India Society initiated training for welfare workers to give them skills in working with people. In 1936, a philanthropic trust, the Tata Trust, initiated training in professional social work by founding the Tata Institute of Social Sciences.

Today, India has several colleges which provide professional training in Social Work. Social work in the country embraces two primary approaches. First, the welfare and charity approach is practiced by many social work practitioners and non-governmental organizations. This is considered a traditional model of social work practice where the social worker is considered the giver of services and the recipient is a marginalized or poverty stricken person/family or suffering from trauma. Second is the rights-based approach to social work practice. From this perspective, deprivation, marginalization, and human suffering are seen as violations of human rights as enshrined in the Indian constitution. Thus social work practitioners help in providing for clients' needs, while recognizing that the client has a right to this need being fulfilled and the social worker has a duty to help the client fight for these rights. This perspective motivated the Right to Information Act, the Right to Education Act, the Child Sexual Abuse Act, and many government policy and program changes.

A Social Worker Responds

Ben belongs to the middle class whereas Marang belongs to the poor class. In India, Marang would belong to the Scheduled Caste (defined previously as the "outcastes") and also to the poor class. Being from different castes means that the couple is under tremendous societal pressure to break up. Additionally, the concepts of privacy and individual decision-making are still not common in India, meaning that the entire family, and the community elders, would have been involved in the case by the time it came to the social worker. The social worker will then have to work with the entire family with all the complications that come with multiple opinions and expectations.

A professionally trained social worker in India would first have to get acquainted with the cultural, social, and religious norms of the clients.

Initially, the social worker will take a detailed case history. Since Bonolo approaches the social worker with a request to "help Ben to come to his senses," the social worker will have to gather information as to why Bonolo thinks Ben needs help. This information will enable him/her to formulate an assessment of the situation which will help Bonolo to decide on future action

The social worker will make it clear to Bonolo that even if she and Ben's family expect him/her to convince Ben to leave Marang, he/she will not be able to do so. The social worker will explain that they will play the role of facilitator and enable Bonolo and Ben to decide what they think is best for them. The worker will offer to meet Ben and discuss the situation with him and help him get clarity in his decision making.

As mentioned earlier, faith in spiritual healers is so entrenched in most parts of the country that the social worker will choose not to get into any discussion about the family's visit to the spiritual healer or opinions about Ben being bewitched. This frame is to avoid the discussion veering away from the main goals of the sessions, or the session being abruptly terminated by the family on the advice of the healer if he gets an inkling about the social worker's negative comments about him. At the same time, the social worker will also acknowledge and accept that the family has faith in the healer and will keep a quiet watch to ensure that the healer does not engage in any harmful or exploitative practice. If he/she finds this happening, the social worker will need to contact the educated aunt and seek her help in reducing the influence of the healer on the family.

The social worker will next focus on rapport building and help the client ventilate her frustration and anger. He/she will ask the client to facilitate a meeting with Ben. Depending on his willingness to open up to him/her, the social worker may even attempt to explain to him the social implications of marrying a girl from a different class. The worker will then suggest that he/she will be willing to meet him again in case he wanted to discuss the matter further. If she comes to meet the social worker, Mary will be counseled to give Ben space and not to pressurize him. After the session with Ben, the social worker will have to withstand the pressure from the family to divulge the content of the meeting. It is important to note here that although advice giving is not a preferred practice in professional social work, in the Indian context, clients often do insist on being advised.

In case Ben decides to marry Marang, the social worker will accept it as he/she believes in allowing the client the right of self-determination. He/she will also facilitate the family's understanding of the situation and help Bonolo come to terms with it. Lastly, he/she will show his/her willingness to meet any of them again if they need any further help in the future.

Exercises

Discussion Questions

1 Discuss how issues of spirituality emerge in couples in your country.
2 In what ways do the styles/approaches of conflict management used in solving conflicts between partners differ between countries?
3 To what extent is social work practice with couples in your country evidence-based? What research has been done on intervention with couples in your country?
4 How do you decide which is the best theoretical approach to take in working with couples?
5 What is the best way to deal with clients' traditional beliefs, such as the use of faith healers, which might conflict with the social workers' own beliefs?
6 What are your country's legal or cultural attitudes toward infidelity? How does that impact how you might work with clients?

Classroom Exercises

1 Role play Case Study #5, Ben and Bonolo, having one student serve as the social worker. Then analyze with the whole class: what do they think about the decisions the social worker made? What might each student have done differently or the same?
2 In dyads, students should share their own moral attitudes towards fidelity in partnerships or marriage. In the same dyads, they should then discuss how these attitudes might impact their work with clients. How might their attitudes manifest in counter-transferential responses? What is the best way to work with these feelings?

References

American Psychiatric Association (2008). "Coping with AIDS and HIV." Retrieved from http://www.healthyminds.org/Main-Topic/HIV-AIDS.aspx
Anderson, J., & Doyal, L. (2004). "Women from Africa living with HIV in London: A descriptive study". *AIDS Care*, 16 (1), 95–105.
Anderson, W. (2004). *The needs of people living with HIV in the UK A guide*. London: National Aids Trust.

Ashford, J. B., & LeCroy, C. W. (2010). Human behavior in the social environment: A multidimensional perspective (4th ed.). Belmont, CA, Brooks/Cole, Cengage Learning.

Cairns, G. (2008). "Circumcising HIV positive men may increase HIV infections in female partners but fewer STIs seen." Retrieved from http://www.aidsmap.com/CROI-Circumcising-HIV-positive-men-may-increase-HIV-infections-in-female-partners-but-fewer-STIs-seen/page/1429386/

Cook, J. A., et al (2004). "Depressive symptoms and AIDS-related mortality among a multisite cohort of HIV-positive women." *American Journal of Public Health,* 94 (7), 1133–1140.

Beckett, C. (2002). *Human growth & development.* London: Sage.

Bronfrenbrenner, U. (1979). The ecology of human development: Experiments by nature and design. Cambridge, MA: Harvard University Press.

Casement, P. (1985). *On learning from the patient.* New York: Routledge.

DeFrain, J. (1999). "Strong families around the world." *Family Matters,* 53, 6–13.

Department of Health (2005). HIV and AIDS in African communities: A framework for better prevention and care, London: Department of Health.

Desai, M. (2002). Ideologies and social work: Historical and contemporary analyses. Jaipur: Rawat Publications.

Erikson, E. H. (1982). *The life cycle completed. A review.* London: WW Norton.

Erikson, E. H. (1987). A way of looking at things: Selected papers from 1930–1986. London: WW Norton.

Erikson, E. (1995). *Childhood and society.* London: Vintage.

Eviandaru, M., & Widyatmoko, C. S. (2004). "Membaca problema personal, membaca jati diri komunal (analisa rubrik konsultasi surat kabar harian Kompas)." Proceeding National Simposium APTIK Research 2004. Bandung: Parahyangan Catholic University

Gardner, R. (2002). *Supporting families: Child protection in the community.* Chichester: John Wiley and Sons.

Gore, M. S. (1965). *Social work and social work education.* Bombay: Asia Publishing House.

Health Protection Agency (HPA) (2010). "HIV in the United Kingdom: 2010 Report." Health Protection Report 2010 4 (47). Retrieved from http://www.hpa.org.uk/webc/HPAwebFile/HPAweb_C/1287145367237

Health Protection Agency (HPA), Health Protection Scotland, UCL Institute of Child Health (2011). "United Kingdom New HIV Diagnoses to end of June 2011." Retrieved from http://www.hpa.org.uk/webc/HPAwebFile/HPAweb_C/1237970242135

Health Protection Agency (HPA) (2011). *HIV in the United Kingdom: 2011 Report.* Colindale, London: Health Protection Services.

Her Majesty's Stationery Office (HMSO) (1990). "NHS and Community Care Act 1990." London: HMSO. Retrieved from http://www.legislation.gov.uk/ukpga/1990/19/section/47

Hopson, B., & Adams, J. (1976). *Transition – understanding and managing personal change*. London: Martin Robertson.

Holmes, T. H., & Rahe, R. H. (1967). "The social readjustment rating scale." *Journal of Psychosomatic Research*, 11, 213–18.

Horberg, M. A., et al (2007). "Effects of depression and selective serotonin reuptake inhibitor use on adherence to highly active antiretroviral therapy and on clinical outcomes in HIV infected patients." *Journal of Acquired Immune Deficiency Syndromes*, 47 (1), 384–390.

Howe, D. (2005). *Child Abuse and neglect attachment, development and intervention*. London: Palgrave.

Huntingdonshire Primary Care Trust (2005). Multi-agency prebirth protocol.

Koprowska, J. (2005). *Communication and interpersonal skills in social work*. Exeter: Learning Matters.

Kubler-Ross, E. (1997). *On death and dying*. USA: Touchstone.

Laming, (2003). *The Victoria Climbie Inquiry Report*. HMSO: UK

Moon, J. (2004). *A handbook of reflective and experiential learning: Theory and practice*. London: Routledge Falmer.

Munro, E., & Calder, M. (2005). "Where has child protection gone?" *The Political Quarterly*, 76, 439–45.

Munro, E. (2011). *The Munro review of child protection: final report: A child-centred system*. London: Crown Copyright.

Nelson, T. S. (2010). "Explanation and description: An integrative solution-focused case of couple therapy." In A. S. Gurman (Ed.). *Clinical casebook of couple therapy* (pp. 44–66). New York: Guilford Press.

The National Survey of Sexual Attitudes and Lifestyles (NATSAL) (2001). "Britain Uncovered."

National AIDS Control Organization (NACO) (2008). *HIV sentinel surveillance and HIV estimation in India 2007: A technical brief*. New Delhi: NACO.

NHS and Community Care Act 1990. London: HMSO. Retrieved from http://www.legislation.gov.uk/ukpga/1990/19/section/47

Office of National Statistics (ONS) (2010). Divorces in England and Wales, 2010. Retrieved from http://www.ons.gov.uk/ons/publications/re-reference-tables.html?edition=tcm%3A77-238035

Palmer, G., Carr, J., & Kenway, P. (2005). *Monitoring poverty and social exclusion 2005*. York: Joseph Rowntree Foundation/New Policy Institute.

Parker, R., & Aggleton, P. (2002). "HIV/AIDS related stigma and discrimination: A conceptual framework and an agenda for action." New York: Population Council.

Philips, A. (2007). *Winnicott*. London: Penguin.

Prime Minister's Strategy Unit (2005). *Improving the life chances of disabled people*. London: Cabinet Office.

Probyn, E. (2003). *The spatial imperative of subjectivity*. In K. Anderson, M. Domosh, S. Pile & N. Thrift (Eds.). *Handbook of cultural geography* (pp. 290–99). London: Sage.

Rogers, C. (1951). *Client centred therapy*. Boston, MA: Houghton Mifflin.

—. (1961). *On becoming a person*. Boston, MA: Houghton Mifflin

Ross, H., Gask, K., & Berrington, A. (2011). "Civil partnerships five years on." *Office for National Statistics (ONS)*. *Population Trends*, 145.

St. George's Paediatric HIV Team (2003). Where do I start? Talking to children with HIV about their illness. London: St George's Paediatric HIV Team.

Stinnett, N., & DeFrain, J. (1985). *Secrets of strong families*. Boston, MA: Little Brown.

Stroebe, M. S., & Schut, H. (1999). "The dual process model of coping with bereavement." *Death Studies*, 23, 197–224.

Sudbery, J. (2010). *Human growth and development: An introduction for social workers*. London: Routledge.

United Nations (UN) (2000). United Nations issues wall chart on marriage patterns 2000. Retrieved from http://www.un.org/esa/population/publications/worldmarriage/worldmarriage2000PressRelease.htm

United Nations General Assembly Special Session (UNGASS) (2010). "Country progress report: India." Retrieved from http://www.unaids.org/en/dataanalysis/monitoringcountryprogress/progressreports/2010countries/india_2010_country_progress_report_en.pdf

Wilson, K., Ruch, G., Lymbery, M. & Cooper, A. (2008). Social work: An introduction to contemporary practice. Gosport: Ashford Colour Press.

Worden, W. (1992). *Grief counseling and grief therapy*. New York: Springer Publishing Co.

World Health Organization (WHO) (2003). HIV infected women and their families: Psychosocial support and related issues. Geneva: World Health Organization, Department of Reproductive Health and Research. Retrieved from http://www.whqlibdoc.who.int/hq/2003/WHO_RHR_03.07.pdf

WHO Media centre (2006). Treatment for sexually transmitted infections has a role in HIV prevention. Retrieved from http://www.who.int/mediacentre/news/releases/2006/pr40/en/index.html

Intimate Partner Violence

4

By Caren J. Frost

Domestic violence, intimate partner violence and abuse are terms often used interchangeably (Taft, Broom & Legge, 2004) in reference to acts ranging from violent physical assaults to emotional and psychological abuse, which occur in intimate relationships. Women most often suffer from intimate partner violence. Men are sometimes victims and not always perpetrators; however, male victims are less prone to sharing with others incidents of violence perpetrated against them (Loue, 2001). Though intimate partner violence is considered a problem worldwide (Flaherty, 2010; UNICEF, 2000; WHO, 1996), there are variations in what constitutes this form of violence (WHO, 1996). These differences affect incidence or prevalence estimates. UNICEF (2000) and WHO (1996) indicate that the issue of intimate partner violence is widespread, and despite the unavailability of very accurate statistics, note that between 20 and 50 per cent of women worldwide have experienced some form of this type of violence. There is limited information about male victims. Multiple factors are cited for the numerous incidents of intimate partner violence. Some of the causes are institutionalized and thus considered normal in some societies. In some parts of the world, violence against female partners is predicated on certain social, cultural, and religious norms. Gender, economic hardships, and indulgence in drugs can be factors that account for intimate partner violence in some societies. The information in this chapter will present some "typical" cases and country-specific analyses for each case.

Case study #1

Emotional Abuse/Verbal Abuse in a Marriage

BY JOANNA E. BETTMANN FROM THE US

Dan is a 45-year-old man living in a major city with his wife of 20 years, Sue. They do not have children, but live close to their respective families and enjoy spending time with their nieces and nephews. Dan works as a carpenter and Sue as a house cleaner. Dan and Sue have a rocky marriage, marked by several separations. They have shared many happy moments and both love each other very much; however, Dan struggles to manage his temper, particularly when depressed. His depression particularly emerges when his self-esteem drops, such as when he loses a job or the couple are struggling financially. At these times, Dan becomes verbally aggressive to Sue. He calls her names like "Bitch" and "Whore," tells her she is "worthless," and says "I'm sorry I ever married you."

His name-calling and insults have a significant impact on Sue. She has never thought of herself as particularly capable or talented, but she works hard and enjoys being with her colleagues. When Dan calls her names, she believes him. She begins, at those times, to feel worse about herself and does not challenge him. When he yells at her, she simply says, "Dan, please don't" in a quiet voice, and she'll ask, "What did I do wrong?" Because Dan's verbal aggression comes from his own depression (rather than being prompted by something Sue did), his responses are always confusing to her. She experiences his verbal aggression as suddenly here and then suddenly gone. She doesn't know how to prevent it or help it; she simply tries to survive the onslaught of name-calling and insults when he gets upset.

Although she loves Dan deeply, Sue has contemplated leaving the marriage. Several times in the last ten years, she has gone to live with her sister for many weeks after an especially brutal verbal tirade. Every time, though, she ends up concluding that she loves Dan, that she's getting older, and that it is likely no one else would want her. After Sue's most recent stay at her sister's house, her sister encouraged her to speak with a social worker who had been helpful to Sue's sister and her husband in working through their marital conflicts.

Emotional Abuse/Verbal Abuse in a Marriage: A Social Worker from Ghana Responds

BY AUGUSTINA NAAMI

Prevalence and Incidence

Widespread domestic violence is a global phenomenon; Ghana is not an exception to this trend. Studies show that, in Ghana, one in three women suffers physical violence from a past or current partner, three in ten women experience sexual abuse, and 27 per cent experience psychological abuse (Corker-Appiah & Kusack, 1999).

Country Policies

The idea that marital issues are a private matter is being demystified. The existence of a domestic violence law, a Domestic Violence and Victims Support Unit of the Ghana Police Service, and a Commission on Human Rights and Administrative Justice indicates that abused women can seek redress outside a family which seems to be dysfunctional.

The Commission on Human Rights and Administrative Justice (CHRAJ) (1993) responds to fundamental human right abuses, including domestic violence, and is enshrined in the Constitution of the Republic of Ghana. CHRAJ responds to human rights abuses through negotiation, mediation, panel hearing, and court action, where necessary.

The Domestic Violence and Victims Support Unit, on the other hand, is a branch of the Ghana Police Service responsible for handling issues regarding domestic violence. The unit, which was formerly called the Women and Juvenile Unit, was established in 1998 and seeks to prevent and protect against, as well as prosecute, perpetrators of domestic violence. The unit handles matters concerning marital, custodial and maintenance issues and provides counseling and supportive services to victims of abuse.

The first legislation to specifically address domestic violence in the country is the Domestic Violence Act (732) (2007). The law provides protection for women against all forms of abuse—physical, sexual, economic, and psychological—within an existing or a previous relationship. Once an incident is reported, an arrest is made after a medical report confirms the act. The case passes through the judiciary system and a protection order is issued depending on the situation.

A Social Worker Responds

Three factors can be attributed to domestic violence in Ghana: traditional beliefs, economic dependence/independence, and customary practices (Cantalupo, Martin, Pak, & Shin, 2006). Ghanaians see women as inferior to men and hence expect women to submit to men, particularly their husbands, at all times, irrespective of the decisions that ought to be made (Coalition on Women's Manifesto for Ghana [CWMG], 2004). Decision-making in marriage is solely a man's responsibility, since he is considered the head of the household.

The extended family system is another traditional belief. Ghanaians believe that anything that affects a family member affects everyone else in the family; hence family members do everything to help preserve the good name of the family. There is also a belief that domestic violence is a private family matter and should be handled within the family. Seeking redress to domestic violence outside the family is equivalent to "washing one's dirty clothes in public." Families, therefore, try to ensure that all family issues are resolved within the family.

Other contributory factors to domestic violence are economic dependence, where women depend on their husbands for their livelihood, and economic independence, where women have other sources of income. Some Ghanaian men see the latter as a threat to their control over the household. Finally, customary practices, where men pay an expensive bride price (payment from the groom's family to the bride/bride's family), contribute to domestic violence. Some of the tribes accept an exorbitant bride price, a practice that makes men feel they have bought the women and, hence, can do whatever they please with them.

These beliefs compel female victims to accept domestic violence and discourage them from reporting it. Reporting abuse formally might result in the collapse of a marriage since it could create tension within the family. In some instances, when abuse cases are reported formally, family, church, and traditional leaders intervene to withdraw the case in favor of an amicable out of court settlement (Cantalupo, Martin, Pak, & Shin, 2006).

The social work profession, though relatively old, struggles to gain recognition in Ghanaian society in comparison to other professions. In the past, social workers were seen as welfare officers, mediating between the government and the vulnerable population. However, the profession is currently emerging, with many social workers engaged in other settings including hospitals, prisons, community development programs, marriage and family settings, and child welfare services.

Regarding the current case, the social worker will let the woman know she is safe with him/her and that the social worker can be trusted. Efforts will be made to ensure that the woman is comfortable so that she can express her feelings about the situation. It is important that the social worker find a private place to discuss the issue because, due to the lack of office space in Ghana, many offices are shared. It is important to let the woman know that she did not do anything to cause the situation, and that she is not the only person experiencing the problem. However, the woman must also know that it is wrong for her husband to call her names or yell at her. His behavior is unjustified and unacceptable.

The social worker and the woman will work to identify her coping mechanisms, affirm the strengths she already has and explore more options to manage the situation. The social worker will inquire if the woman has a religious preference since Ghana is recognized as a religious country with 69 per cent Christian, 16 per cent Muslim, and 9 per cent traditional believers (Central Intelligence Agency, 2010). If she has a religious preference, they will together map out faith-based activities that could help the woman's situation. Other coping mechanisms are laughing (to herself) at some of the things the man says and thinking positive things about herself when the man tries to make her feel worse and calls her names.

The social worker will refer the woman to domestic violence social support networks. An example is the Gender Violence Survivors Support Network (GVSSN), a resource to meet and discuss her problems openly with other abuse survivors.

The social worker will also use assertiveness and confidence building techniques alongside the coping training identified earlier. He/she will begin by helping the woman to recognize her capabilities and talents, so that she will stop thinking negatively about herself. He/she will also let the woman know that ignoring her husband's behavior all the time does not help to manage the situation. The woman must learn to discuss the issue with her husband. In Ghana, it is said that the best time to discuss marital problems is at dawn. The woman could wake her husband at dawn and express her feelings about what had happened the previous day. She will be taught the importance of talking about her feelings, and at the same time being respectful of the husband so that he does not get hurt in the process and become angrier and more aggressive. The social worker will teach the woman assertiveness skills, emphasizing the importance of using "I" statements to communicate her feelings. For example, "I am hurt when you call me a bitch. Please don't do that. I have a name and would appreciate it if you call me by my name." She will model the statements to ensure she handles them well.

These mechanisms will be used to see how the man responds. If he listens to the woman, that will be a breakthrough, but if he does not and continues to abuse the woman, then it is advisable to include him in the therapy. Based on the new laws, there is a possibility that the man will agree to therapy. If the man does come for therapy, the social worker will begin the process by letting him gain the worker's trust. The professional will find out why the man abuses the woman, for example: Was he brought up in an abusive home? Does he associate with abusers? Is childlessness an issue? The professional will then follow through to find out if he still sees the qualities he saw in the woman before they married. The social worker will work with the man to help him to understand the negativity of his actions, and take him through this assessment process. He/she will find out more about the man's job and the problems he experiences on the job. The social worker will also discuss the family's budget and how it is managed. If the finances are mismanaged, he/she will teach the couple financial management skills. If the man also has a religious preference, he will be encouraged to participate in spiritual activities. Although Ghana has a rich culture, some aspects of the culture contribute to domestic violence and discourage abused women from formally reporting the abuse.

Emotional Abuse/Verbal Abuse in a Marriage: A Social Worker from Mongolia Responds

BY CHANAR GOODRICH

Prevalence and Incidence

Domestic violence is one of the most serious problems for women in Mongolia. It has been hidden for some time in many Mongolian households, because of the high rate of unemployment and increasing alcoholism among rural low-income families. Harsh economic and political transitions from the early 1990s left Mongolian public health and social sectors facing numerous challenges. A research study conducted on the prevalence of physical, emotional and financial violence against women in Mongolia showed that alcohol was associated with all three types of violence (Shagdarsuren, et al. 2009). The increasing number of domestic violence cases caused by alcohol abuse has become an important priority for many non-governmental organizations (NGOs) advocating against violence. Traditional values in Mongolia have begun to disappear. Mongolian society has a tradition of protecting women from violence. According to (Shagdarsuren, et al. 2009), "In the 13th century, Mongolia developed a legal code that severely punished offenders who abused women, who caused pregnant women to miscarry, or who touched personal belongings of women without permission." According to the *Secret History of Mongolia*, the oldest surviving literary work written during the twelfth century about royal Mongol women's influence and power in society, women commanded in war, presided as judges over criminal cases, ruled vast territories, and rejected different customs of neighboring cultures for women such as wearing the veil, binding their feet, or being secluded (Weatherford 2010). In the past, Mongolian men were taught to respect women and provide for their families at a young age. Mongolian culture and tradition is strong in its demand for respect of women and there are many traditional folksongs praising mothers and their unconditional love for their children and mankind. Generally, Mongolian women are not oppressed; however, there is inequality among men and women in areas such as employment benefits, wage disparity, and economic and political opportunities. In the traditional family, the majority of decisions in a marriage involve both husband and wife. On certain occasions, extended family members are included and, depending on the situation, such extended families help raise children if necessary.

Mongolian women who suffer domestic violence may appear more submissive to their husbands, boyfriends and partners out of fear for their children and the shame it could bring to the family. They often hide what is going on in their lives from others. Talking to people, especially strangers, and seeking help with domestic violence issues are not common among survivors. A famous Mongolian proverb might help explain why people don't air their dirty laundry in public: "A broken or cracked bone is better than lost honor or reputation." Victims of domestic violence open up only to their family members and people they trust. It is difficult for social workers to break through the social stigma created by domestic violence in Mongolia.

The lack of public awareness and necessary services for the victims of domestic violence keep Mongolians unaware of the issue. According to the National Center Against Violence (NCAV) the number of domestic violence victims seeking help has increased from 29 in 1995 to 729 in 2008. A 2008 NCAV study considered the social factors contributing to domestic violence and determined that, out of 78 domestic violence victims involved in the study, 53 reported that violence occurs when the perpetrator is drunk. In addition, 68 per cent reported that they are abused only at home, 18.6 per cent in the workplace, 7.4 per cent in the homes of others, while 6 per cent reported being abused by their spouses or partners in public places.

The government-supported shelters available to victims of domestic violence are insufficient. Without government support and a basic foundation of social services, Mongolian domestic violence victims will continue to suffer the consequences of violence through their partners' verbal and physical abuse. Since domestic violence is perceived as a family dispute, government legislators have done little about this issue in Mongolia. Even though there is little support or training from the Mongolian government, there are many NGOs that are concerned about women and children who are victims of domestic violence. According to the US Department of State's Country Reports on Human Rights Practices (2003), there were no reliable statistics regarding the extent of domestic abuse; however, the NCAV estimated that approximately one in three women is subject to some form of domestic violence and one in ten women is physically battered.

Country Policies

Although Mongolia has a 2004 law against domestic violence, the law does not provide a clear definition of domestic violence. No amendments have been made to other relevant laws following the domestic violence legislation; therefore, the safety and protection of victims still remains in question. Although the Mongolian government Policy on Public Health, officially adopted in 2002, states that it is a requirement to "establish a favorable psychological environment for families, communities, and society as well as preventing and combating violence," little or no improvements have been made on reducing alcohol abuse and domestic violence issues. Despite the existence of government policy statements, however, reports and studies from NGOs show different results regarding high rates of alcoholism and domestic violence. According to the NCAV, the court has issued only 22 restraining orders since the domestic violence legislation came into force. Due to a lack of systematic training programs, law enforcement officers have little awareness about the law. In 1992, Mongolia passed the Law on Administrative Liability, which governs assault and misconduct under the influence of alcohol. Law enforcement officers apply this law instead, neglecting the real danger that the victims are facing with domestic violence. According to NCAV, 2,415 out of 9,114 people detained in 2006, with 1,179 out of 4,979 detained in first half of 2007 detained, according to court verdicts, due to domestic violence. In 2006, 4,728 out of 8,683 people were detained, while in the first half of 2008 2,102 out of 4,107 people were detained according to the Law on Administrative Liability. Applying this law to domestic violence cases causes more dramatic victimization to the victims. Since they do not approach domestic violence as a crime, police and law enforcement organizations put it last on the priority list and the police do not intervene unless the perpetrators are drunk. The drunken perpetrators are taken to the sobering house and are required to pay for the service. The basic fee for the sobering house is 4,150 MNT (about US $4), but this often reaches 7,900 MNT (about US $7.50) including additional services. Victims also have to pay 10,000–12,000 MNT (about US $11) for sending their perpetrators to the sobering house.

There is no other known police, governmental social agency, or law enforcement intervention in domestic violence cases. The head of the general police department of Mongolia approved a procedure on administrative sanctions in 2004 (order No. 139) which states: "Administration of the detention center shall organize meetings with family members or relatives more than once a week for up to three minutes for detainees." This procedure does not help protect victims of domestic violence, but further victimizes and traumatizes them.

A Social Worker Responds

The concept of "social work" is new to Mongolia. People often view social workers as distributers of foreign aid. Social workers in Mongolia lack proper education and training to help people, specifically victims of domestic violence. Since the perception of domestic violence is that it is a family affair, social workers experience difficulties in intervening in these situations. However, through media and news items, survivors are beginning to understand the importance of seeking help, even though they have limited options when attempting to do so on their own.

The job of the social worker is to cooperate with local hospitals and law enforcement agencies to aid survivors. It is important for social workers to let people know that help is available and to educate them on relevant issues. Educating the public about the social work profession is the key to intervention in cases of domestic violence. Social workers need to have a safe haven for survivors to speak about their issues so that they are encouraged to seek help. Thus social workers must exude confidence in order for the victim to understand that seeking help is not shameful. Education on domestic violence and how those involved are able to overcome their fears needs to be the focus of training for social workers in Mongolia.

Delivering domestic violence interventions can be tricky in Mongolian society, as people often live together as couples without being married. Due to the gray areas in legal definitions of domestic violence, there is a lack of public and professional understanding about what it entails.

Physical and Psychological Abuse within a Partnership

BY TIRELO MODIE FROM BOTSWANA

Teko is a 28-year-old woman from a rural, remote village. She attended primary school, but no secondary school. She is currently unemployed. She has one child with an ex-boyfriend whom she no longer sees. She met her current boyfriend, Sedimo, aged 30, at a bar nine months ago. Sedimo is unemployed and spends most of his time drinking at the bar. On several occasions, he has beaten Teko, saying he suspected her of cheating on him.

The most violent beating occurred when he found her at the bar talking with another man. He shouted at her, kicked her, and punched her with his fists all over her body. The beating was so violent that she fainted. The next day she was hospitalized due to internal wounds from the beating. Since the beatings began, she is unable to bath herself due to her wounds. She is frequently bruised all over, from her face to other parts of her body.

She says she wants to leave him, but he is refusing to terminate the relationship. On several occasions he has threatened to kill her if she left him. Because of these beatings, Teko often fails to perform her household chores or even take care of her child properly. Sedimo has told her not to associate with her friends and even some of her relatives, explaining that he needs to be the most important person to her. Consequently, Teko has not talked to her family, who live several hours away, in many months. Teko states that she is consumed by thoughts of the suffering she has experienced at the hands of Sedimo. Her life is untenable and yet she feels totally disempowered and unable to change her circumstances. One of Teko's friends at the bar encourages her to talk to the social worker who visits their local health clinic on a monthly basis.

Psychological Abuse in a Relationship: A Social Worker from Mexico Responds

BY NARCEDALIA PRATT CORNEJO

A Social Worker Responds

Arroyo Grande, Guerrero, Mexico is a town with a population of about 500 inhabitants. The town does not have a police station, but there is a major city nearby (a two-hour bus ride away). I am not an expert on the criminal justice system in Mexico, but I have observed how people take justice into their own hands.

Abuse is hard to report in Mexico, especially in a small town. Many such towns do not have a police station so if someone wants to press charges against another; the person has to take the bus to a big city with a police station, paying about U.S $2 for bus fare. It is a difficult process to press charges against someone for physical abuse. Women turn to their mothers and friends for support, but are told time and again to stop making their spouses upset and be obedient. Obedience consists of having dinner on the table when he walks in the door, not questioning their husbands' affairs, and by participating in sex whenever the boyfriend/husband wants it.

The people in the village do not consider emotional abuse as being abuse. Women in Mexican small towns do not see physical abuse as a bad thing; they see it as normal and/or even something they bring upon themselves. Since many women are homemakers, they typically go to the market each morning to purchase groceries for the day. A large number take this outing as an opportunity to talk to other women (family and friends) at the market. Women can go to the market with bruises and a black eye and others will not question this because they already know that the person's husband hits her. Law enforcement is absent so this avenue is often not an option. On occasion the city's mayor gets involved after harassment by the townspeople to intervene, but this situation does not happen regularly. As an example, on one occasion a husband beat his wife and she had bruises but no broken bones. The abuse gradually escalated to a point where the wife was left unconscious. She was taken to the city the following day with several broken ribs, a dislocated arm and a broken nose. The city's mayor became involved. The townspeople were afraid the husband was going to kill her if no one intervened. The spouse did end up going to jail and his wife moved out of the state due to fear of his return and/or retaliation.

I grew up in Mexico and lived there until I was ten years old. I visited the country in 2009 after the death of my father. Many people remember me, and came to my grandmother's house to visit. The visitors asked me on several occasions if my spouse treated me well, and if he hit me. They did not believe that my spouse did not hit me. Emotional abuse was never brought up; women talked more about their need to be good spouses hoping that their spouse would not hit them so often.

Emotional abuse is not considered abuse among the village people, but the Mexican government is trying to educate people about abuse through television commercials. Abuse is much better handled in big cities where law enforcement agencies are present. If a woman reported emotional abuse in the big city, the police would probably not open a case because they would want to see evidence—but how can one prove emotional abuse? Physical abuse is, however, punishable by law in bigger cities.

As another example, a friend of one of my siblings was severely abused in Mexico. The woman was beaten by her husband to a point where he broke her nose and a couple of ribs. Her family was not supportive; they told her to stop being so demanding. She was admitted to a hospital and questioned about what happened to her but she denied any physical abuse. Her husband had threatened her in the past, saying that if she ever tried to put him in jail he would take the children and she would never see them again. Months later she was admitted to a hospital again with serious injuries. This time she reported what happened and her husband went to jail. Social services only provided her with a referral to receive psychotherapy services. This woman lost her children because her husband's family took them into hiding and threatened her. She immigrated to the US where years later she met and married what she thought was a good man. He physically abused her and would threaten to end her immigration application (to get her green card). She endured the abuse until she obtained her green card and then she left him. Two months later she found out that she was pregnant but never told her ex-husband due to fear that he would take away her baby.

Psychological Abuse within a Partnership: A Social Worker from India Responds

BY HENA JOHN-FISK

Prevalence and Incidence

In India, domestic violence cuts across all ages, religions, castes, education, and economic circumstances. Females are taught to accept, justify, bear, and keep silent about any kind of violence, especially domestic violence, due to shame, fear, and family honor. According to the National Crime Report

Bureau, every three minutes there is a crime perpetrated on a woman, every 29 minutes a female is raped, every 77 minutes a woman dies because of dowry disputes, and every 9 minutes a woman faces cruelty at the hands of a husband and/or relatives (BBC, 2006). According to the UN Population Fund Report, approximately two-thirds of married Indian women are victims of domestic violence and as many as 70 per cent of married women in India between the ages of 15 and 49 are victims of beating, rape or forced sex (Press Trust of India, 2005).

Country Policies

In 1983, the Indian government declared domestic violence an act of cruelty at the hands of husbands or family members under section 498-A of the Indian Penal Code. This law had many loopholes; for instance, all female police stations and counseling cells were supposed to be set up across the country but implementation was limited to urban areas. The law did not address violence happening in homes, especially between husband and wife. Since there was no separate civil law to address domestic violence, there was no protection and rehabilitation available for battered women and punishment and imprisonment was not the best solution. After a long and constant fight with NGOs, the Indian government amended the existing domestic violence law to pass a much more comprehensive law known as the Protection of Women from Domestic Violence Act (2005). The new law did not meet all of the expectations of non-governmental organizations, but was welcomed. Some of the main features addressed by this new law included marital rape, rehabilitation, and protection for women, as well as protection orders against husbands and live-in partners who abuse women emotionally, physically, or economically.

A Social Worker Responds

In this case study, Teko is a 28-year-old female who is a victim of domestic violence and is socially isolated. Her boyfriend, Sedimo, has restricted her to only having one friend. The first thing a social worker would do is to complete an intake sheet with Teko's details like name, age, religion, home address, employment, and history of violence. Under the Protection of Women from Domestic Violence Act (2005), anyone who is aware of domestic violence may report this incident to a protection officer, magistrate, or police officer. It should be noted that it is not mandatory for an organization or a person to report an act of violence (Protection of Women from Domestic Violence

Act 2005). Only if she gives consent can the organization file a woman's report with the police. Teko's case can be handled in two different ways depending on her decision about filing a report with the police.

If Teko chooses to file a police report against her boyfriend, then the organization would accompany her to a police station. In India, a female victim is the only person who can file a First Information Report (FIR) with the police. She could be accompanied by a family member, friend or an organization representative. The police would file a report against Sedimo under the Domestic Violence Act. This act protects married women or females in a live-in relationship from domestic violence. In terms of this act, Sedimo would be arrested and then prosecuted under the law. He could be imprisoned for a year, have to pay a fine of US $450 or both.

Under this act, the protection officer or service provider could request medical benefits from medical facilities for Teko. She could be taken to a government hospital for a medical examination. The copy of the medical report would then be given to the police officer and magistrate. The non-profit organization would help Teko with her medical expenses and keeping a regular follow-up appointment with the doctor. Teko would be accompanied by the medical social worker on every hospital visit she makes in the future. Teko's responsibility would be to pay half the travel cost to the hospital and half the medication cost. If she is unable to pay, the organization would attempt to get monetary assistance for her.

In line with the conditions of the assistance, Teko would be enabled to meet her expenses due to losses she suffered because of violence. Teko could get a protective order which would prevent her boyfriend from coming close to her at her residence, office, or any place commonly visited by Teko and her child's school. He would also not be able to access their joint bank account. Apart from the above, Teko could get shelter under this act. The magistrate can order any shelter to provide protection for Teko. We should note that India does not have specific shelter homes for victims of domestic violence. Teko could also get a residence order that would secure the right to housing in the same apartment/house where she was residing with Sedimo, even if she does not own the house or if the lease is not in her name. Along with these benefits, this act would provide legal aid and counseling services to Teko from any relevant organization. The organization would do everything under the act to provide the benefits to her. It would also provide individual and group counseling for Teko. If needed, she would be referred to a psychiatrist by the psychologist in the organization.

Since he threatened to kill Teko, Sedimo could be prosecuted under the Indian Penal Code Section 307 for an attempt to murder. He could be imprisoned for up to ten years or life if Teko is harmed (Indian Penal Code, 1860). Additionally, the organization working with Teko could report Teko's case to the National Commission for Women, which would provide her with legal aid (National Commission for Women Act, 1990).

This scenario would be different if Teko decided not to file a police report against Sedimo. She most likely would make this decision if she is scared that he will harm or kill her or her children. The social worker would ask Teko to have a medical examination to find out if she needed medical attention. If Teko changes her mind in the future, she could use this examination to file a police report against Sedimo. The organization will help her with her medical bills and in that case she will pay ten Rupees (less than half a US dollar) for the medical papers for the government hospital, and also pay half the cost of travel to the hospital.

After the medical examination is completed, the medical social worker would go through the details with Teko, such as when to take her medication and when to have a follow-up with the doctor. The medical social worker would report the details to Teko's case worker. After this, Teko would meet the organization's psychologist/counselor; she may also need to meet a psychiatrist if the counselor refers her. The counselor and the social worker will know all the details of her case and they would maintain confidentiality in that regard. She would receive individual counseling in the initial phase and group therapy if she desires it.

In the individual session, the counselor would build rapport. She/he would not force Teko to share her story. Only when Teko is ready would she do so. After hearing her story, the counselor would give several suggestions to Teko who would solely decide what she wants to do in her particular situation. For instance, the counselor would offer her the options of shelter, job opportunities, skill building workshops, child care information, relationship related workshops, or filing a police report.

If Teko chooses to act on all of the options, she will be helped in the following manner: since she has not filed a legal complaint she would not get access to government shelter home facilities under the Protection of Women from Domestic Violence Act. In her case, the organization can help her find accommodation in a non-profit organization's shelter home. There are a number of government and non-governmental hostels available for women. Survivors can also take shelter in a reliable family member or friend's home.

If Teko already has a job, and if her boyfriend harasses her at work, then the non-profit organization can work with Teko's employers to keep her boyfriend away from the office premises. Since she has not filed a report with the police, she cannot obtain a protective order. Another option could be asking the employer to transfer Teko to a different location, which could be a risky action to take since her boyfriend could get angrier with her and do her more harm. Before taking this step the counselor would discuss the possible effects of this action with Teko. The counselor could also combine this option with obtaining housing before taking this step. Another option would be applying for a new job. If Teko needed a job, child care, or skills training, then the organization would refer her to different organizations which could help her meet her various needs.

If Teko expresses the desire to get help with her relationship, then the counselor would design specific sessions on relationships. The counselor would also refer her to support groups where she could talk to different women who are victims of domestic violence. These are some of the services the organization would provide to Teko other than increasing her sense of awareness and education about domestic violence. The organization would help Teko with legal aid if she expressed the desire to file a report against her boyfriend. If Teko changes her mind and files a police report, her case would be handled according to the Protection of Women from Domestic Violence Act and/or the Indian Penal Code, section 307. These are some of the ways physical and psychological abuse cases can be handled by social workers in India.

Case study #3

Sexual Violence in a Marriage/Partnership

BY CAREN J. FROST FROM THE US

Amanda met Bill when she was 19 years old. She was a single mother, and Bill, who was handsome and funny, had a good job and showed interest in her. At first, Amanda did not feel any attraction to Bill. In fact, she felt overwhelmed by his attentions and flattery. He sent flowers and bought her attractive gifts. Eventually he convinced her that he was the man for her and they moved in together in her small house.

Once living together, Bill began to make comments about other women that Amanda felt were crude and mean. He became possessive of her and told her she should not talk to men without his permission. Amanda began to make excuses for his behavior with her friends and family—saying he was overworked but was a good provider for her and her three-year-old daughter.

Bill became increasingly hostile and then violent toward Amanda. When he later apologized for his behavior, Bill said it was because he had had a terrible childhood and been abandoned by his mother when he was six years old. Bill said he was afraid that Amanda would leave him and that is why he was so possessive.

As their relationship continued, Bill asked Amanda to marry him, which she did in part because Bill convinced her that no one else would have her. Once Bill began to tell her that she was not very good in bed, Amanda began to believe that too. Amanda thought that because Bill was her partner she had to give in to his need for violent sex, even if it hurt and led to serious injury to her. She was frequently covered with bruises on her arms and legs from their rough sex.

Amanda's friends stopped supporting her, because she spends all her time trying to make Bill happy so that he will not hurt her. One night after they had been married for a year, Amanda declined to have sex with Bill and he proceeded to rape her repeatedly. In subsequent months, Bill called Amanda names and told her that she was a whore who does not know good sex when she is getting it.

Bill always apologizes for hurting Amanda, but she has begun to believe he is not sorry and that he will never change. Bill frequently threatens to kill Amanda if she tries to leave. She is terrified that Bill will kill her and her daughter, who is now five years old. Amanda thinks she wants to leave Bill, but does not know how. One day a friend comes to see Amanda while Bill is at work. The friend brings a female social worker who deals with violence against women to meet Amanda.

Sexual Violence in a Marriage/Partnership: A Social Worker from India Responds

BY SHARVARI KARANDIKAR

Prevalence and Incidence

Domestic and sexual violence is widely underreported in India. Recent statistics indicate that between 10 and 14 per cent of married women are raped by their husbands: the incidents of marital rape soar to one-third and then to one-half among clinical samples of battered women. Sexual assault by one's spouse accounts for approximately 25 per cent of rapes committed. Dowry is still the most common cause of violence against women in India. Even though India has legally abolished the institution of dowry, dowry-related violence is actually on the rise. More than 5,000 women are killed annually by their husbands and in-laws, who burn them in 'accidental' kitchen fires if their ongoing demands for dowry before and after marriage are not met.

Country Policies

The policies on preventing violence and helping victims are limited in India. The Domestic Violence Act of 2005 considers violence and sexual abuse against women as a criminal offence. However, the law is not implemented and women are often reluctant or scared to use the legal system for help in marital relationships. Provisions such as government shelters, counseling and medical services are available for victims but they are limited to urban areas and few women are able to take advantage of them.

A Social Worker Responds

Social work organizations working on domestic and sexual violence use either individual case work or family intervention for helping victims. Social work organizations also work closely with law enforcement agencies to ensure that perpetrators of violence are arrested and legal help offered to victims. Although laws in India protect the victims and penalize the perpetrators, the domestic violence law is seen as the last option in a relationship. Female victims of violence try to work on their relationship and save the marriage—taking police action against their husband is the last resort. Due to this reason, family intervention is more effective. A social worker in a family intervention setting would talk to the victim but also to the perpetrator and other family members involved in the situation. There would be several individual meetings with the victim and the perpetrator, followed by joint meetings where they are encouraged to communicate and rationalize their differences. The goal of family intervention is reconciliation given that family and marriage are important institutions in India. However, in cases of severe violence and physical and mental health problems, victims of violence are provided with several resources and legal action may be taken against the perpetrators. All decisions are made in consultation with the victim.

In Amanda's case, a female social worker would set up an appointment to meet in her office or any other safe location for Amanda. In the first meeting, the social worker discusses her role as helper and facilitator. She assures Amanda about confidentiality and briefs her about the process of counseling and family intervention. The four steps involved in family intervention are: meetings with the client, meetings with the perpetrator, joint meetings with client and perpetrator, and follow-up meetings. The social worker informs Amanda that, although the aim of family intervention is reconciliation, in some cases it is safer for the woman to end the relationship. The social worker informs Amanda that if she decides to end her relationship with

Bill she will be provided with help through women's shelters, legal aid, and women's self-help groups in the nearby community. The four steps of family intervention are discussed below.

The first meeting between victim and the social worker is the in-take interview meeting where Amanda would describe the nature of her problem and reasons for approaching a social worker. The social worker fills out an in-take form and listens to Amanda. She may take notes and ask questions for clarification. At this stage, the social worker also tries to establish rapport. She may encourage Amanda to talk, reinforce confidentiality and demonstrate empathy to ensure that Amanda feels safe in disclosing her problems.

The consecutive meetings with Amanda are more structured and the social worker asks more questions about the client's s recent experiences of violence. She may also explore Amanda's feelings of guilt, self-pity, and helplessness in order to understand her view of her marriage. If Amanda is blaming herself for the violence, the social worker confronts her beliefs. Amanda is made aware that it is not acceptable for the husband to beat and rape his wife. The social worker may refer Amanda for psychological screening and help if she feels that she is depressed and needs additional support. She also takes into account other family members who may be important to Amanda regarding marital decisions. In this case, Amanda's daughter and her care may be discussed at length by the social worker. During these meetings, the social worker provides resources such as alternative living options for Amanda and her daughter and/or discusses the possibility of her living temporarily with a family member. Amanda is given specific tasks at the end of each meeting which may involve refusing to give in to Bill's demands, communicating with Bill about his abusive behavior, protecting herself from abuse, reporting violence to the police or informing a family member or a helpful neighbor.

After a series of individual meetings with Amanda, the social worker discusses whether she wants to go ahead with family intervention and involve Bill in the counseling process. If Amanda agrees to family intervention, the social worker invites Bill to participate in the counseling process. However, if Amanda feels she does not wish to continue her relationship with Bill, the social worker provides her with guidance for filing for legal separation.

Family intervention requires the social worker to meet Bill and talk to him about his marriage. The social worker explains to Bill that she has been helping Amanda to cope with the violence, and provides him with an opportunity to discuss his point of view and his feelings about the marriage. Since Bill is suspicious of Amanda and possessive of her, the social worker discusses his fear about the marriage and encourages Bill to seek psychological help. She informs Bill that, unless he changes his behavior, Amanda would not be able to live with him. She recommends that Bill seek therapy and monitors whether there is any behavior change after a period of time.

Joint meetings are arranged with Amanda and Bill. The social worker clearly states all the behavior changes that were agreed upon by both Bill and Amanda and, over the next few weeks, the social worker monitors whether any incidences of violence are reported by Amanda.

If the situation improves, counseling is terminated and Amanda and Bill return for follow-up sessions. However, if there is no significant improvement in Bill's behavior, Amanda is given the option of seeking legal help which can range from taking police action against Bill to filing for separation and divorce. This option is typically stressful for women in India. A lot of stigma is attached to separation and divorce and women find it difficult to live independently. Often, other family members are invited by the social worker to intervene and help the victim. The social worker networks with other agencies providing shelter, employment and children's education to help Amanda. The social worker works with lawyers for her to gain custody of her daughter and to help Amanda to interpret the law.

This model of social work intervention for domestic and sexual violence is seen in the Special Cell for Women and Children in Mumbai. This unit works with the Mumbai Police Department, and social workers are located in offices in police stations around Mumbai. When they approach the police to complain about violence from their husbands, women are referred to the social workers. The social workers follow the above-mentioned family intervention model to help victims. Through this method, victims get police protection from their abusive husbands, and in some cases their in-laws and other abusive family members. The victims also have access to legal aid though the Special Cell and all services are offered free of charge.

Sexual Violence in a Marriage/Partnership: A Social Worker from Ghana Responds

BY PETER DWUMAH & LISA SALMA ABUBAKAR

Prevalence and Incidence

Sexual violence in marriage is just one in a range of abusive acts people in marital relationships in Ghana face. Prior to revisions in Ghana's criminal code and the passing of the Domestic Violence Bill in 2007, there were no provisions that allowed for charges to be brought against husbands for forcibly having sex with their wives. Even with the passage of the Domestic Violence Bill and the review of the Criminal Code that resulted in the criminalization of marital rape, the whole idea or concept of marital rape is considered absurd by most Ghanaians, men and women alike. The new provisions allow for the prosecution of men who have sex with their wives without the latters' approval (Archampong, 2010; Ghana Demographic and Health Survey, 2003).

Generally, information about the prevalence of sexual violence in marriages and relationships in Ghana is based on casual observation. Literature showing empirical reports on such matters is lacking and there are few studies with reports on sexual violence in marriages and relationships. In 1998, a study was conducted with a total sample of 3,047 people (females 66 per cent and males 34 per cent). Eight per cent of the females reported having had an experience of forced sex, and 5 per cent of the males had forced sex on their partners. Fifty-nine per cent of the people affected indicated they made no reports of their experiences to anybody; an indication of how such issues remain unreported or underreported (Ardayfio-Schandorf, 2005). The results of a more recent survey involving 11,778 households indicate that 8 per cent of women had experienced sexual violence from a spouse or partner (Ghana Statistical Service (GSS), Ghana Health Service (GHS), and ICF Macro, 2009).

A Social Worker Responds

With reference to the case of Amanda and Bill, in Ghanaian traditional society a woman is subordinate to a man and whatever the man says must be done. It is said that the woman is expected to "satisfy the man in bed," meaning to satisfy the man sexually. So in Ghanaian traditional culture, there is nothing like rape in marriage. As married couples, any time the man demands sex, the woman should be willing and avail herself to him. This expectation is influenced by the notion that, in Ghanaian traditional society, a woman does not contribute economically. It is rather the man who does everything and therefore the woman has no say in relation to the demands of the man. It is assumed that the man owns the woman, because of the rites performed by the man. For instance, some tribes pay cattle as the bride price which allows a man the right to a woman's reproductive capacity.

In contemporary times, women are more assertive and their rights are recognized. A man cannot have his way if he maltreats a woman. Government agencies such as the Department of Social Welfare and the Domestic Violence and Victim Support Unit (DOVVSU) of the Ghanaian Police Service are there to safeguard or protect women from sexual violence indicated in the case involving Amanda and Bill. This safeguard is backed by the Domestic Violence Act (Act 732) (2007).

With regard to the current case involving sexual violence in marriage, first the social worker needs to investigate the situation to appreciate the problem. This fact-finding exercise would require background checks on the couple, as well as interacting with both Amanda and Bill, colleagues, relatives, and others. In Ghana, this case can be seen by the social worker as a criminal case, because there is an element of criminality with reference to the Domestic Violence Act. The Act states that a person in a domestic relationship who engages in sexual violence or rape commits an offence and is liable, on summary conviction, to a fine of not more than 500 penalty units, or to a term of imprisonment of not more than two years, or both.

The social worker in Ghana will plan an intervention strategy to help save Amanda and her daughter. Bill's frequent threat to kill Amanda should give the social worker the basis to report this case to the police for his arrest. The interest of the victim is paramount to the social worker, who has to assist Amanda in deciding what she wants. Should Amanda and Bill show interest in reconciliation, the social worker will have to counsel them on healthy patterns of communication and help both of them to deal with Amanda's wounded feelings. Bill will need help managing his aggressive behavior and sexual habits.

If the social worker reports this case to the police for prosecution, the court can grant a protection order based on the interest of the clients. The social worker who is the probation officer will observe Bill and report on his subsequent conduct to the court. If the appointed social worker or probation officer reports that he has engaged in any act of sexual violence after the settlement, Bill shall be brought before the court and prosecuted, possibly facing a term of imprisonment of not less than one month and not more than two years or both, or not more than three years for the contravention of the protection order.

With reference to the divorce, the action of the social worker would depend on the type of marriage arrangement in which the clients are involved. Marriages are contracted by customary, ordinance, and Islamic means. Customary marriage entails the performance of just the traditional marital rites. In this case, the social worker would counsel Amanda to ascertain the process of divorce from her family since there are variations in the process of divorce depending on her ethnic origin. Marriage by ordinance entails the performance of customary rites as well as the involvement of the church. The Islamic marriage follows Islamic principles. In these types of marriages, the social worker would help Amanda make her own decisions regarding divorce.

Exercises

In Class

The following exercises are for in-class discussion. Please remember that not all your peers will have the same views as yours on these issues. Being able to explore these issues together and discuss them in a supportive environment is crucial to obtaining a better understanding of intimate partner violence.

- Describe what you would do if you were the social worker for any one of these cases. Compare how that response would be different from/similar to the responses provided. Why would your response be different from/similar to the responses provided?
- Consider the role of law enforcement agencies in incidents of intimate partner violence. Are there cultural parameters that constitute a hindrance as to how law enforcement agencies respond to incidents of intimate partner violence? How do social workers and law enforcement agents work together in your home country when these issues occur?
- How are male survivors and non-heterosexual victims of intimate partner violence protected in your home country? Why is this the case? What does this mean for some vulnerable populations who experience violence?

Outside of Class

For each of the exercises below, select a country different from your home country and the countries discussed in this chapter. Be prepared to present your findings to your peers in class.

- Search for sources in another country that provide information about intimate partner violence. Summarize what the resources are and where they are located.
- Consider the laws in another country that deal with intimate partner violence. Compare the laws to those in your home country. Who do the laws protect? Why?
- Conduct a thorough literature search about the impact of extended family members on rates of intimate partner violence in one or two countries. Draft a summary about the information you find on this topic.
- Develop a list of agencies in your country that could support victims of intimate partner violence. What are the mission statements of the

agencies? How are the statements linked to actual practice for social workers?

- Interview one or two of your social work peers about their knowledge of intimate partner violence in another country. Ask him/her about the incidence of and community attitudes toward intimate partner violence. [Do not get into a debate about the issues—uncover facts and/or information based on opinions only.]

References

Archampong, E. A. (2010). Marital rape – A women's equality issue in Ghana. Faculty of Law, KNUST, Kumasi, September, 2010.

Ardayfio-Schandorf, E. (2005). 'Violence against women: The Ghanaian case'. Retrieved from http://www.un.org/womenwatch/daw/egm/vaw-stat-2005/docs/expert-papers/Ardayfio.pdf

BBC (2006). 'India tackles domestic violence'. Retrieved from http://news.bbc.co.uk/2/hi/6086334.stm

Cantalupo, N., Martin, L. V., Pak, K., & Shin, S. (2006). 'Domestic Violence in Ghana: Open secret'. *Georgetown Journal of Gender and Law*, 7, 531–592.

Central Intelligence Agency (2010). Ghana: Population, religion. Retrieved from https://www.cia.gov/library/publications/the-world-factbook/geos/gh.html

Coalition of Women's Manifesto for Ghana (CWMG) (2004). *Women's Manifesto for Ghana*. Accra, Ghana: Combert Impressions.

Corker-Appiah, D. & Cusack, K. (1999). 'Breaking the silence & challenging the myths of violence against women & children in Ghana: Report of a national study on violence.' Accra, Ghana: Gender Studies & Human Rights Documentation Center.

Flaherty, M. P. (2010). 'Constructing a world beyond intimate partner abuse'. *Affilia: Journal of Women & Social Work*, 25 (3), 224–35.

Ghana Statistical Service (GSS), Ghana Health Service (GHS), and ICF Macro (2009). *Ghana demographic and health survey 2008: Key findings*. Calverton, Maryland, USA: GSS, GHS, and ICF Macro. Retrieved from http://www.gendercentreghana.org/article_details.php?id=10

Ghana Statistical Service (GSS), Noguchi Memorial Institute for Medical Research (NMIMR) and ORC Macro (2004). *Ghana Demographic and Health Survey 2003*. Calverton, Maryland: GSS, NMIMR, and ORC Macro.

Indian Penal Code, 1860. Retrieved from http://www.indianlawcases.com/Act-Indian.Penal.Code,.1860-1759

Ley de Asistencia Social (Law on Social Welfare), D.O. Retrieved from http://www.diputados.gob.mx/

Loue, S. (2001). *Intimate partner violence: Societal, medical, legal and individual responses*. New York: Kluwer Academic/Plenum.

National Commission for Women Act, 1990. Retrieved from http://ncw.nic.in/ frm ABTMandate.aspx

Oyunbileg, S., Sumberzul, N., Udval, N., Wang, J-D., & Janes, C.R. (2009). Prevalence and risk factors of domestic violence among Mongolian women. *Journal of Women's Health 18(11)*, 1873–1880.

Press Trust of India (2005). Two-thirds of married Indian women victims of domestic violence: UN. Express India. Retrieved from http://www. expressindia.com/news/fullstory.php?newsid=56501

Protection of Women from Domestic Violence Act, 2005. Retrieved from http:// indianchristians.in/news/images/resources/pdf/protection_of_womenfrom_ domestic_violence_act_2005.pdf

Taft, A., Broom, D., & Legge, D. (2004). 'General practitioner management of intimate partner abuse and the whole family: qualitative study'. *BMJ (Clinical Research Ed.)*, 328, 618–21.

UNICEF (2000). 'Domestic violence against women and girls'. Innocenti Digest. Innocenti Research Centre, Florence, Italy. Retrieved from http:// www.unicef-irc.org/publications/pdf/digest6e.pdf

US Department of State Country Reports on Human Rights Practices for 2003. Retrieved from https://www.internationalrelations.house.gov/archives/ 108/92389vI.pdf

Weatherford, J. (2010). The secret history of the Mongol queens: How the daughters of Genghis Khan rescued his empire. New York: Crown Publishing Group.

World Health Organization (1996) 'Violence against women'. WHO Consultation, Geneva: WHO. Retrieved from http://whqlibdoc.who.int/ hq/1996/FRH_WHD_96.27.pdf

<table>
<tr><td>5</td><td></td></tr>
</table>

5 | Family Conflict

By Gloria Jacques

The family is the basic unit of society. It is regarded as the primary agent of socialization and plays a very important role in the formative years of each individual. Although the significance of the family is widely recognized, there is no single definition for what it is. Over the years the conception of what a family is has evolved, and customary notions of familial relationships and institutions have been affected by advancements and developments in societies around the world (Lamanna & Reidmann, 2006; Weigel, 2008; Wilson, 1985). During the life course, family members develop implicit beliefs related to themselves (as individuals and as members of the family system), their environments, and their world view or family paradigm. Traumatic life stressors, such as illness, death, or incarceration, for example, require the family to change its mode of functioning and integrate a new reality into their world view. In the process, the family group may transform itself and create a new paradigm (Germain & Gitterman, 1996). The reality of culture and the new paradigm creates shock waves affecting the individual, nuclear and kinship groupings, the community, and society as a whole. The cases and analyses in this chapter illustrate the variety of issues families face and how they deal with these changes.

Case study #1

Working with a Dysfunctional Family

BY JOANNA E. BETTMANN FROM THE US

Maria and Ned are a married couple in their early 30s who have three children (ten, seven, and four). They have been a couple ever since they were 16, and they are each other's primary support. Maria has not talked to her family in years. She was raised in a home with an extremely abusive, alcoholic mother and a father who was away at work in the oil fields for months at a time. She and her four siblings never became particularly close—they competed for attention and affection from both unavailable parents. Ned, on the other hand, maintains a fairly close relationship with his family. He talks with his mother at least several times a week and enjoys taking the children to her house to play. Ned's father died of cancer when he was eight.

Maria works as an office assistant for a factory manager, but recently her job situation has become tenuous. The factory is making fewer goods, since there is less demand for the goods overseas. Thus, workers at the factory are beginning to lose their jobs. Maria is worried that she will lose her job in the near future. Ned's job is similarly in jeopardy. He works as a pharmacist at a local store, but the store was recently bought by a large conglomerate which is restructuring, eliminating some positions, and reassigning some workers. Ned and Maria are under stress and they have begun to fight frequently.

Maria tells Ned that she does not like how much time he spends with his mother. She says that it is wrong for him to pay so much attention to his mother and that he does not pay enough attention to her. Ned tells Maria that she does not spend enough time with him or the children, that she spends too much time on things that do not matter such as buying things for the family, watching television, and visiting friends. Both have begun drinking more than usual and their fights have become loud. Occasionally, Ned and Maria will push each other, but usually they just shout. Neighbors have complained to the police about the yelling and last weekend the police came to the house demanding that they quieten down. At that point, the oldest child emerged from her bedroom and told the policeman that her family was fine and to leave them alone. The police said that they would only write up the neighbors' noise complaint and that no charges would be filed if the family saw a social worker to begin to work out their issues.

The next week, Maria and Ned come to the social worker's office with their three children. They explain that they have had a long, relatively happy marriage, but recently things have become strained. They say that it is affecting their marriage and perhaps their children and that they need help.

Working with a Dysfunctional Family: A Social Worker from Botswana Responds

BY MOSARWA SEGWABE

Prevalence and Incidence

The results of the Botswana AIDS Impact Survey III (BAIS III) conducted in 2008 showed that 57.7 per cent of the populations aged 12–74 years were never married while 15.7 per cent were married. Only 1.1 per cent of this population reported being divorced. The same study showed that 37.4 per cent of the respondents stated that they had at some time consciously taken alcohol. Of all males aged 10–64, 14.8 per cent took alcohol one to two days in a week, while the comparable percentage for females was 5.1 per cent. The highest proportion of male and female respondents who took alcohol occasionally was 18.5 per cent and 13.9 per cent respectively. BAIS III estimated the overall unemployment rate at 26.2 per cent with females hardest hit (31.2 per cent) relative to their male counterparts (21.9 per cent).

Country Policies

Social work is still a developing profession in Botswana. Academic training provided by the University of Botswana saw the first group of students with a Bachelors degree (BSW) graduate in 1990. Since then postgraduate degrees have been offered at Masters level and, in late 2011, at doctoral level.

The Government of Botswana (GOB), through the Ministry of Local Government (MLG), has the largest social services program in the country. Under the Ministry there are two departments that are responsible for the implementation and coordination of social services: the Department of Social Services (DSS) which is responsible for policy, legislation, coordination, and capacity building, and the Department of Social and Community Development (S&CD) which is at district or local authority level throughout the country and is responsible for the implementation of laws and policies relevant to the programs that fall under their area of operation

Current interventions provided by the MLG include social care and protection programs related to orphans and vulnerable children, destitute persons, and families in need of assistance at all levels. Social workers implementing these programs are deployed throughout the country as the GOB plan is to ensure that even people in the remotest parts of the country are provided with social services. These social workers often multi-task, work with minimal resources, cover extensive geographical areas, and address competing priorities while receiving minimal supervision.

A Social Worker Responds

A social worker in Botswana would immediately concentrate on the job issue, providing counseling to help the couple process their anxiety related to the possibility of job loss and to make them realize how the anxiety is creating other problems such as tension, excessive alcohol use, and poor parenting. The worker would help the couple to explore their lives in detail, looking particularly at their financial situation including their spending patterns and their debt situation. This process would be aimed at helping the clients to think about how best to organize their lives to minimize the impact of one or both of them losing their jobs. The worker may opt to refer them to a financial planner, provided they are able to pay for such services, or to their bank. The counseling that the social worker provides would also be aimed at preparing the couple to emotionally and psychologically deal with the possibility of job loss in the family. It would also concentrate on helping them to communicate (in an assertive manner) their feelings and thoughts so that they would be able to appreciate each other's situation and provide support.

The social worker would then focus attention on other issues such as alcohol use and abuse. Even though the couple started drinking heavily after they began experiencing problems at work, it does not necessarily mean that everything will automatically normalize once the work situation has been addressed. The helper would encourage the couple to explore their reasons for drinking and provide the necessary counseling, focusing on the consequences of excessive alcohol intake, and helping them to formulate a plan to wean them from their alcoholic tendencies. In a country like Botswana, where HIV prevalence is 17.6 per cent among the general population, it would be critical for the social worker to address issues related to HIV and AIDS and how excessive alcohol consumption may place one at risk of acquiring the virus. A population-based study on alcohol and high-risk sexual behaviors in Botswana conducted by Weiser et al., (2006) showed that heavy alcohol use was associated with higher risk of all sex-related outcomes including unprotected sex, multiple sexual partners, and paying for sex. If they continue to drink, the social worker would keep working with them and, if they are in the cities of Gaborone or Francistown, refer them to the Alcoholics Anonymous support group or Lifeline for further intervention.

Once progress has been made with the couple, the social worker would involve the children in the counseling process, helping the parents to share what they are going through with them. The children in this case are old enough to recognize when things are not going well at home, but they are also too young to know how to deal with the situation. This confusion can affect them negatively in relation to school performance and their confidence in relationships with other children. It is important that the children understand what is happening and are provided with the necessary support. Thus the social worker would help the couple to communicate effectively with their children. This process may be difficult for the parents because generally, in Botswana, children are excluded from issues that affect the family; they are considered too young to understand and some families do this with the positive intention of protecting the children.

The social worker should always keep in mind the fact that Maria has no relationship with her own family. Family is important in social work interventions since it is seen as a critical support system or possibly a major source of dysfunctionality. The people of Botswana view family as a critical support system. For example, in the event of death, members of the immediate and extended family would leave their homes for up to two weeks and congregate at the home of those experiencing the loss to provide support. This support is also apparent in the case of children who have lost their parents. Families in Botswana do not believe in sending orphaned children to institutional facilities; they tend to take the responsibility of raising the children in home settings in a demonstration of support and love. In the absence of this kind of system, Maria may not always have the people that she needs around her to help her to cope. Furthermore, Ned is very close to his family, to a point where Maria is now complaining about it. She does not have what Ned has, hence she may not understand how important that support is for Ned, especially at this difficult time in his life. The social worker would discuss this with the couple, helping them to understand how different their lives are in terms of the assistance they receive from their families of origin. This discussion would, hopefully, help Maria to understand how significant it is for Ned to maintain contact with his mother. At the same time, the social worker would work with Ned to help him realize that Maria does not have what he has and that he (and hopefully his mother) should be there to support her at this difficult time in her life.

Working with a Dysfunctional Family: A Social Worker from Japan Responds

BY KAYO TOBINAGA

Prevalence and Incidence

Problems related to alcohol abuse, depression, and sleeping disorders are social concerns in Japan. It is common for work-related stress to be brought into the home, especially since the proportion of employed persons is very large. It is not unusual for Japanese people to give priority to work rather than time spent with their families and friends. Life expectancy, at 83 years, is the highest in the world (World Bank, 2009). On the other hand, the suicide rate per 100,000 is very high, at 36.5 for females and 14.1 for males (World Health Organization [WHO], 2008). The number of suicides in 2009 was 31,690 people, and included high numbers of unemployed men in their fifties (Japan National Police Agency, 2009). Workaholic tendencies and death from overwork are also issues of concern. The rate of unemployment is 4 per cent (World Bank, 2009) and numbers of temporary and contract workers are increasing although traditionally lifetime employment has been the common trend.

Country Policies

Japan's population is estimated at around 127.7 million (The World Bank, 2009) and its society is linguistically and culturally homogeneous with a small population of foreign workers. Health care services are provided by national and local government, and payment for personal medical services is offered through a universal health care insurance system that provides relative equality of access, with fees set by a government committee. There are child welfare consultation centers and public health centers which offer free access to social workers for the public in every city, and some companies have contracts with industrial counselors who can offer free psychotherapy services. "Social worker" is a general term for social workers and psychiatric social workers with government certification.

A Social Worker Responds

A social worker would find potentially positive aspects that would help to solve the problems in this case. In Japan, it is not often that the husband comes for help since couple counseling is not common. When all come for help together it means that they all recognize that they have a problem and need to share their feelings and, significantly, have the motivation to address related issues. Maria and Ned have had a long, relatively happy marriage and history of working. It shows that they have the social skills to maintain family functioning if all things go relatively well and they do not have serious personality problems. Their dysfunctional family history is recent, and they have not lost interest in the functionality of their family.

It is thought that the main problems in relation to this family's dysfunction are anticipatory anxiety, fear, and work-related stress of the parents. Both are anxious concerning employment in the near future, although they have not lost their jobs yet. It is very hard to find employment after losing a job through restructuring; therefore, the anxiety of losing a job can be a cause of stress especially for someone who has young children.

Clients can be considered to be struggling with unresolved issues from the past and remembered personal experiences can be regarded as influential factors that keep individuals "stuck" in their own idiosyncratic world views that guide them in their relationship. In terms of Ned's history, he had the tendency to take care of his mother from childhood. He used to care for her and puts a high priority on being together with his family. Concerning Maria, she was raised in an abusive family and has not prioritized spending time with her family members. This priority gap between Maria and Ned might be one of the causes of conflict. Obviously their fighting in front of the children might be affecting the children's mental health and they might feel too guilty to visit their grandmother's house. Furthermore, this issue would affect the social life of the children such as friendships, school performance, and relationships. Generally, they may not be able to concentrate on anything while experiencing family difficulties.

There is more violence when people consume alcohol because they are less in control of their feelings and behavior. Maria and Ned might drink to forget their problems, but this is not a solution. On the contrary, drinking creates unnecessary conflict in their family since it develops dependence on alcohol rather than helping them to face their problems.

First of all, a social worker in Japan would organize a family session where all members can talk about their problems. Individual sessions would also be arranged and the social worker would organize sessions for the children with a psychologist to assess the effect of the problems on them. If the social worker needs information from the children's class teachers, he/she could obtain a report from them with the permission of the parents. Social workers would make an assessment of the family's problems and share this with the parents. The anxiety and fear attached to loss of employment would be acknowledged, but they would be reminded that they have not yet lost their jobs. No one can tell whether they will be confronted by that challenge, but it is very natural for people who have responsibility for taking care of children to have such a fear. Furthermore, anxiety acts as a signal that psychic danger would result if an unconscious "wish" were to be realized, meaning that the parents are unconsciously preparing to face the coming challenges. Explanation of the nature of anxiety would help the parents to be calmer and to rethink problems from another perspective.

The social worker would ask the parents about their stress management strategies, including what they do or who helps them when they are stressed. It seems that this couple uses alcohol as a coping mechanism, and the family appears to be in a vicious spiral that might be affecting family life as a whole. Generally, stress is not a cause but a reaction to the pressure that people feel. Social workers would try to identify this pressure and give them positive options to deal with their stress in a more constructive way. They would also teach them strategies to help them cope with the stress, such as breathing and relaxation techniques and anger management strategies.

It is extremely common in Japan for clients to view struggles in a "linear" or "blaming" context. The philosophy underlying this context is that there is one basic reason for a problem and one sole cure. The problem is being created by something, or someone, and if the specific cause could be uncovered, a solution would become readily apparent. Maria and Ned seem to be blaming each other and trying to find the *cause* of family issues when ideally they should be helping each other to face the challenges. Ned used to take care of his mother after his father died, and Maria might not understand the reason why he still cares so much since she grew up in an abusive family. On the other hand, Maria used to solve most of her problems on her own since she was not able to count on her own family. When people become stressed, they tend to use the strategy they have previously chosen in their lives. Every family member has their own character and life history and it is natural that there are priority gaps and divergent tendencies. Furthermore, Maria and Ned have managed to maintain a relatively happy marriage for quite a long time and to cope with many challenges. Social workers would explore this situation with them and identify related strengths and resources.

In preparation for facing the challenges, the social worker would give them practical information about the labor law in Japan whereby the employer needs to inform their employees in advance if he/she plans to dismiss them. Also, employees cannot be fired without sufficient reason, in which case they can refuse to leave. The client can seek help from the labor union, a lawyer, or the labor office free of charge. Even if they lose their job, they would be paid a severance allowance and unemployment insurance for a year. In Japan, there are government employment agencies (called "hello work") in every city and they offer free services related to all labor issues. This kind of practical and realistic information would help the clients to prepare to face the challenges without unnecessary fear.

Case study #2

Parental Illness in a Family

BY BOITUMELO MALEBOGO SEGWABANYANE FROM BOTSWANA

Felistus was a 40-year-old refugee living in a new country of resettlement. He had two children with a cohabiting partner, Tiny, also from his country of origin, who had two children of her own aged 15 and 17. Felistus was a builder by profession but had been unemployed for several years. He occasionally got work as a day laborer in neighboring villages.

Several years ago, Felistus went for an HIV test at the local clinic. He tested positive. Tiny never tested but always promised to do so. She said that she knew she was HIV negative. Last year, Felistus fell ill. Doctors discovered that he had cancer of the eye. They recommended drug therapy for his HIV, as well as chemotherapy for his cancer. However, he was unable to pay for private treatment and could not access government assistance to pay for the treatment he needed. He approached various non-governmental agencies to ask for financial support but they were unable to assist. He finally received drug therapy for his HIV infection from a church group near his home.

Tiny was supportive of him and stood by him during the pain he endured due to the cancer. He never received cancer treatment, however, and his body started to deteriorate. Tiny began having difficulty in engaging in a sexual relationship with Felistus. She disclosed to their home-based care nurse that his odor repulsed her and the children. The house they lived in had only one bedroom and their two elder children began to sleep away from home with neighbors and friends. The two younger children, aged six and nine, started doing poorly in school and bed-wetting. Felistus and Tiny had never discussed his illness with the children but his deterioration was obvious.

Six months ago, Felistus's condition worsened. On bad days, worms crawled out of his eye. Nurses in the local clinic complained that other patients were having a problem sitting in the same waiting room with him because of the smell. Some weeks later he died.

A week after his death, Felistus's relatives chased Tiny out of the home that she had shared with Felistus, saying that she was an illegal immigrant and should return to her birthplace. Social workers discovered that Tiny had been staying in the country illegally for over ten years. She had no travel documents and was faced with potential deportation. She and Felistus were not married and humanitarian agencies were unable to help her. She quickly moved in with a local man and left all the children in the house she used to stay in with Felistus. After being pursued by the authorities to take the children with her and threatened with charges of child neglect, she moved them into her new home. Nine months later, she had a child with her new partner. Issues in this blended family are simmering and the children are confused and unhappy. The older children are struggling in school and not wanting to live at home; the younger children are confused and upset. A child welfare social worker visits the family.

Parental Illness in a Family: A Social Worker from Canada Responds

BY NUELLE NOVIK

Prevalence and Incidence

The case study highlights a number of specific issues, including the impact of HIV and AIDS and cancer. However, the individuals deemed to be most at risk are also impacted by issues related to immigration, and more specifically, by child welfare concerns. As such, the prevalence and incidence of these particular issues in Canada will be explored in more detail.

The adult male in this case study faced two separate life threatening illnesses: AIDS and cancer, the second of which ultimately brought about his untimely death. In Canada, it was estimated that in 2009, there were approximately 68,000 people living with HIV and AIDS, and just over 1,000 individuals had died from the disease. In that same year, the estimated adult prevalence rate of HIV infection was 0.3 per cent (IndexMundi, 2011a). Aboriginal persons are overrepresented in the epidemic and in 2009 comprised 11 per cent of all new infections (Public Health Agency of Canada, 2009). In 2007, cancer surpassed cardiovascular disease as the leading cause of death in Canada (Canadian Cancer Society, 2011). Based on 2011 estimates, 40 per cent of Canadian women and 45 per cent of Canadian men will develop cancer during their lifetimes. Further to this, it is estimated that one out of every four Canadians will die from cancer (Canadian Cancer Society, 2011).

As indicated earlier, this case study also presents issues related to immigration. Increasingly, immigration has become an important component in Canada. According to Statistics Canada (2003), immigration represents close to 70 per cent of population growth, up from 20 per cent in 1976. According to the 2001 Census, 18.4 per cent of Canada's total population is composed of immigrants (Statistics Canada, 2003). There is no credible information available which documents numbers of illegal immigrants in Canada, but 2007 estimates suggest that these range between 35,000 and 120,000 (Ottawa Citizen, 2007). This case study focuses specifically on concerns related to child welfare. In 2007, there were an estimated 67,000 children in out-of-home care across Canada (Mulcahy & Trocme, 2010).

Country Policies

The most pressing policy area to be considered in this analysis is child welfare and, due to potential impact upon the children, current policy regarding common-law marriage is also significant. Provincial and territorial jurisdictions in Canada have legislative responsibility for child welfare except that the federal government has responsibility for Aboriginal peoples with status under the Indian Act (Human Resources and Skill Development Canada [HRSDC], 2000). Child and family service legislation reflects both the scope of involvement of relevant authorities as well as a more holistic approach to assisting and supporting children in need of protection (HRSDC, 2000). Any criminal proceedings resulting from investigations into child abuse and neglect are prosecuted under the Criminal Code of Canada (HRSDC, 2000).

Common law marriages are unions that are not licensed by government authorities in Canada. However, the legal definition and regulation of common-law marriage falls under provincial jurisdiction. According to Revenue Canada (2007), a person with whom you share a conjugal relationship will be considered to be your common-law partner only after your current relationship with that person has lasted at least 12 continuous months. If the common-law spouse dies, the surviving spouse is entitled to pension and survivor death benefits (Canadian Bar Association [CBA], 2010) and if the spouse dies without having drawn up a will, the survivor is still entitled to a share of the estate. In addition, any natural or adopted children are also entitled to a share of the estate under the Estate Administration Act (CBA, 2010).

Finally, it is also important to consider the role of the social worker when considering this case study. An important role of social work in Canada is to support and facilitate the social well-being and functioning of the person-in-environment (Canadian Association of Social Workers [CASW], 2008) and social workers are expected, particularly, to be culturally sensitive and value ethnic diversity.

A Social Worker Responds

At a very basic level, the child welfare social worker in Canada would focus primarily on ensuring the well-being and safety of the children. Initial calls are all received, and responded to, by an intake worker. The intake worker will assess the situation and determine what type of intervention is required. If a child is in imminent danger, the social worker will respond immediately. However, if the child is not deemed to be at immediate risk, the social worker will work with the family by designing a unique approach to connect them with appropriate resources within the community (Ontario Association of Children's Aid Societies, 2010).

Individual provinces and territories in Canada follow their own guidelines and standards based upon legislation specific to each jurisdiction (Government of Saskatchewan, 2010). Responses to a report of child abuse would include the following options: a decision to take no further action, a decision to refer the family to community support services, or a decision to investigate further due to substantiated claims of potential danger to the child (Government of British Columbia, 2007).

Within Canada, a basic principle of child welfare legislation is that the child should be protected and maintained in his or her own home, if at all possible (Government of British Columbia, 2007; Government of Saskatchewan, 2010). If this is impossible, removal of the child is necessary until the family is able to resume their responsibilities to the child. The child welfare social worker is expected to work with the child, parent/guardian, extended family members, and other relevant people to develop a plan which identifies the immediate protection concerns and outlines the strategies for resolving them. This plan also includes a permanency plan which would be put into action if the protection concerns cannot be resolved within set timelines, although all service planning efforts should be focused upon assisting parents/guardians to resume their parental responsibilities as quickly as possible. If this is not possible, other more permanent measures such as private guardianship, permanent guardianship, and/or adoption are considered (Government of British Columbia, 2007; HRSDC, 2010).

The social worker would interview the child in a neutral setting and, if necessary, a police officer should be present. All other children in the home should also be interviewed to determine whether they are also in need of support (Government of Alberta, 2005; Government of British Columbia, 2007).

In this particular case, it would appear that the children may have been experiencing neglect which is defined as a failure to provide for a child's basic needs and involves an act of omission by the parent or guardian (Government of British Columbia, 2007). Behavioral indicators, such as the ones described in this case, may result from phenomena in the child's life such as divorce, separation, or death of a significant person (Government of British Columbia, 2007).

With a focus upon connecting this family to appropriate community support services, Tiny and her new partner would be encouraged to attend counseling or group classes to build healthy communication and co-parenting techniques and strategies. Options for the children would include grief counseling or general support counseling services; peer counseling support that might be available through their schools; and tutoring to assist them in gaining more control over their learning and educational goals. Many social service agencies across Canada also offer structured grief support options including after-school programming, and summer camp opportunities at no financial cost to the family. Tiny and all of the children would also be encouraged to engage in community-based cultural activities that would help them to reconnect with, or remain connected to, their ethnic background. A social worker in Canada would advocate with and on behalf of this family access to their rightful share of Felistus' estate. In this particular case they should be entitled to access to the home that they shared with Felistus or to financial proceedings from the sale of that home. The social worker would also assist Tiny to obtain Canadian citizenship.

Parental Illness in a Family: A Social Worker from South Africa Responds

BY MARGO VAN RENSBURG

Prevalence and Incidence

The growing number of refugees in South Africa contributes to increasing pressure on its resources. This pressure has led to sporadic xenophobic outbreaks by citizens in order to protect their positions. According to Citterio (2010), South Africa is currently the highest single recipient of asylum seekers in the world. He states that, in 2008, the United Nations High Commissioner for Refugees registered more than 207, 200 individual asylum seekers. The majority of these came from Zimbabwe (122,600), Malawi (18,160), and Ethiopia (11,350).

Country Policies

Social workers in South Africa's multicultural society deal, on a daily basis, with the challenges of networking between different languages and cultural groups, including those from neighboring countries. Added to this, they have to find ways of coping with heavy workloads and minimal resources. The Refugee Act (No.130 of 1998) provides for freedom of movement within the host country as well as a right to seek employment, although refugees find it extremely difficult to match their skills and qualifications to job opportunities in the country. Some of the difficulties experienced include lack of language proficiency, limited financial resources to sustain prolonged job hunting, and lack of legal personal documents to obtain work and residence permits. Refugees often have to resort to applying for jobs in the informal sector while their professional skills go untapped.

HIV in South Africa continues to be a social and economic problem and a drain on medical resources. Social workers, HIV and AIDS clinics, and counseling services provide the necessary information, medication, and support for those who have been diagnosed with the illness and for family members needing information. Social workers in South Africa are encouraged to be sensitive to the plight of refugees, and not to discriminate in any way regardless of language, culture, or gender. Since 1998, refugees have had the same rights to access health care as South Africans but, despite this, many feel discriminated against. Non-governmental organizations state that refugees often do not have adequate access to health care. This lack is particularly detrimental for those who are diagnosed as HIV positive and in need of continuous antiretroviral (ARV) medication.

A Social Worker Responds

The case study of Felistus and his family highlights the problems of unemployment, deficient health services, and lack of housing in developing countries. Employment positions particularly are at a premium in South Africa. Although Felistus was a qualified builder in his home country, it would have been difficult to find employment as a refugee. Parental illness in a family affects all its members. According to Manicom (2010), family members as caregivers have also been identified as being at risk of experiencing physical exhaustion and /or emotional stress and burnout. These can lead to increased stress in the home, financial worries through loss of income, absence of a parent while in hospital, and dealing with the side effects of the illness, such as different smells and behavior changes.

The social worker assessing this family would start by conducting a comprehensive assessment of the situation. Interviews would be held with family members, the school, friends and neighbors, and possible religious and aid institutions. When all the information has been put together, the problems can begin to be analyzed and prioritized. Any actions taken will first be discussed between the social worker and relevant family members to determine their suitability and to ensure cooperation between relevant parties. In this case, the most pressing problem appears to be Felistus' HIV treatment and his need for some form of income to support his family. Other problems include Felistus' legal status in South Africa, the changing behavior of the children, and the relationship with his partner.

In most African cultures, details of parental illness are not discussed with the children. Although children may realize there is a problem, it is not verbalized. This silence serves to protect the children from worrying about something they can do nothing about. It is seen as a sign of respect to the children not to burden them unnecessarily.

The position of sharing one bedroom between six people is unsatisfactory. Besides the lack of privacy, these crowded living conditions predispose the development of illnesses and cross infection. The children's safety and welfare are compromised in this case. By not wanting to sleep at home, they are placing themselves in danger of being attacked or possibly raped outside the home, unless suitable alternative living arrangements can be made. The social worker would investigate possibilities of alternative accommodation for the family or a children's shelter where they could be temporarily housed.

Felistus' partner, Tiny, would be advised by social workers to undergo an HIV test to confirm her health status. If she tested positive, she would be encouraged to visit the closest HIV and AIDS counseling and treatment center. Social workers would advise Tiny to legalize her position and apply for refugee status in her own right to avoid deportation after Felistus' death. Moving in with a man and falling pregnant would not give Tiny the automatic legal right to stay in the country. She would have to follow procedural steps to legalize her stay.

The South African Constitution protects the human rights of every person in the country but stipulates the protocol for legalizing the stay of refugees. With refugee status, Tiny would be able to apply for aid from the

Social Relief of Distress Fund. This fund provides temporary assistance for a three-month period, after which re-application can be made.

Applying for refugee status is a lengthy process and, if it is refused, the applicant has 30 days in which to leave the country or lodge an appeal. Because the family disintegrated after Felistus' death, child welfare workers were asked to assist. Social services would reassess the situation and focus on the well-being of the children and Tiny's legal position. They would watch for signs of child neglect both emotionally and physically.

If the children were found to be staying alone and unaccompanied, social workers would consider them to be in need of care and they would be dealt with according to the provisions of the Child Care Act of 1991. The children would be brought before the Children's Court for an inquiry into their personal circumstances. If they were not welcome or were unhappy staying with Tiny's new partner, temporary foster care could be applied for via the courts. It is the policy of social workers and the legal system that children should remain in the care of a parent, as a rule, as long as this is in the best interests of the child.

Parental illness in a family where there are minor children has wide ramifications. From a social worker's point of view, it requires a multi-agency team effort to ensure the welfare of all. The process becomes more involved when the families are refugees. The legal system and social work agencies, however, make it possible for adequate care to be provided.

Case study #3

Effects of Parental Incarceration on Children

BY KGOSIETSILE MARIPE FROM BOTSWANA

Rose is a single female, aged 25, from a small village. She has been incarcerated for the past seven months and still has to serve three more years. She is in her eighth month of pregnancy and about to deliver her baby. She wants help with raising the infant while in prison and also assisting her other child, Nat, aged five, who is currently staying with her aunt.

Rose was convicted of the attempted murder of her son, Nat, and sentenced to prison for five years. Rose says she desperately wants contact with Nat now and regrets her behavior. She says her circumstances forced her to take such drastic action. She states that she was poverty-stricken and without means of support and felt that she had no other option but to kill the child as she was unable to provide for him. She was living with a boyfriend who is the father of the second child. The father of the first had not taken responsibility and threatened to beat her if she revealed his identity.

Although Rose can have visitors monthly, each visit is only 20 minutes long. This visitation time is not sufficient for building parent-child relationships, attachment, or bonding. The visits cannot facilitate development of mother-child trust and warmth. However, it may be unhealthy for Nat to be growing up apart from his mother. Rose's aunt, with whom he is living, is struggling to find ways of explaining Rose's circumstances to him. She is also unsure what role she should be taking with Nat: caregiver, mother figure, something else? Further confusing Nat is the fact that people in the community often say mean things about Rose. These comments are baffling for Nat, who still loves his mother and wants to be with her. Rose was referred to the social worker by the clinic matron while she was serving her term in a women's prison.

Effects of Parental Incarceration on Children: A Social Worker from India Responds

BY HENRY PODHUTASE

Prevalence and Incidence

In India, the attempt to murder is a crime that falls under Section 307 of the Penal Code. Generally, in the prison population, men are in the majority (95.9 per cent) whereas women constitute only 4.1 per cent of the total number of inmates (Prison Statistics of India, 2009). There are a total of 15,406 female inmates in Indian prisons. Among 1,374 such institutions in the country, 18 are specifically for women while the rest have a separate block allocated for females. One of the most difficult situations is that of children who live with their mothers in prison because they lack proper care and amenities for development. Among the women convicts, 469 are living with their 556 children and 1,196 women under trial live together with their 1,314 children (Prison Statistics of India, 2009).

Country Policies

The constitution and laws pertaining to women and children are designed in such a manner that they should receive maximum protection and care from the legal system. The constitution states that children should be given opportunities and facilities to develop in a healthy manner and in conditions of freedom and dignity and that childhood and youth are protected against exploitation and against moral and material abandonment. Additionally, various laws pertaining to women and children, such as the Juvenile Justice Act of 2000, are aimed at providing the best possible protection under the law. In this case, if the client is convicted of attempted murder, she could face up to ten years imprisonment with the added possibility of a fine.

A Social Worker Responds

The social worker will initially open a case file for Rose prioritizing the needs of the client. Later, strategies will be developed to meet these needs. The foremost priority would be to ensure that Rose is treated well in prison. As a matter of immediate attention, she will be provided with emotional and psychological support by the social worker and due consideration would be given to the fact that she is pregnant and should be given appropriate prenatal education. As she might be experiencing emotional turmoil, relevant pre- and post-natal care would be made available for her. Rose can keep her newborn baby with her during her prison term since the Supreme Court of India has given a uniform guideline regarding the custodial care of children in that female prisoners will be allowed to keep their children with them in jail until the latter attain the age of six years.

After creating initial rapport with the client, the worker would inquire about the family and work with Rose to contact them and attempt to reestablish her relationship with them. In this process, Nat's current custodian, his aunt, would also be involved. The worker would discuss with family members various possibilities of care that could be given to Rose at the time of her delivery and would educate her relatives regarding the importance of familial support in her current circumstances. Discussion about the care and protection of Nat would also take place in order to formulate appropriate solutions. All family suggestions would be discussed with Rose in order to help her make an appropriate choice. Based on this outcome, the worker would make the final decision about the person in whose custody Nat should be placed. Options of foster or institutional care would also be considered, but under specific cultural conditions of a collective community (as in India), primary importance would be given to family members as potential custodians.

The social worker would collaborate with NGOs working in criminal justice institutions to support the custodial family of Nat with basic food and health expenses. Additionally the social worker would discuss with Rose the issue of Nat's father and motivate her to file a case against him under the Indian Evidence Act 1972. Under the provisions of the Act, the legitimacy of the child could be ascertained through DNA testing. Even if the father does not want to care for his son, Rose could obtain financial support from him on a monthly basis. The social worker would avail free legal services for her from one of various women's welfare organizations.

The next level of intervention by the social worker would be to develop a strong and loving relationship between Rose and her son through arranging for special sanctions other than the routine 20-minute visitor's time slot. As Rose has to serve three more years, the worker would monitor and help to improve the relationship between mother and son. During sessions with Rose and Nat, the worker would specifically address issues such as neighbors gossiping about Rose, the need for a good relationship between mother and son, and the building of a positive relationship between Nat and the new baby. Nat's case would also be referred to Childline India, which is supported by the ministries of Women and Child Development and Social Justice and Empowerment, for monitoring the care and protection provided by the custodial guardian.

The social worker would also work toward Rose's rehabilitation. Women in India find it more difficult to reenter society after imprisonment than men; however, this is a significant part of the process in the present case. The worker would also collaborate with the prison authorities in appropriate vocational skill development, so that the client would be equipped to find a job after her release. He/she would also work with rehabilitation centers in the client's area of residence to develop a societal reintegration plan for Rose.

Effects of Parental Incarceration on Children: A Social Worker from the US Responds

BY DERRICK TOLLEFSON

Prevalence and Incidence

It is estimated that nearly two million children have a parent incarcerated in prison or jail and that there are 809,000 parents in prison at any given time in the US. In 2007, one in 43 (2.3 per cent) American children had a parent incarcerated in a state or federal prison. Seventy five percent of women and 65 per cent of men in prison are parents (National Resource Center on Children and Families of the Incarcerated, 2011; Mauer, Nellis, & Schirmir 2007). Nearly 10 million children have a parent who is or has been under some form of criminal justice supervision (Hariston, 2004).

Country Policies

In the US, federal law largely dictates child welfare practice. The most pertinent federal law in Rose's case is the Adoption and Safe Families Act of 1997. Under this law, states are required to initiate termination of parental rights proceedings after the child has been in foster care for 15 of the previous 22 months. In rare cases, this requirement can be set aside if it is not in the best interest of the child or if the child is in the care of a relative (Adoption and Safe Families Act, 1997). During this 15-month period the law requires states to make reasonable efforts to provide services to reunite children with their parents. In making decisions about returning the young person to his/her home, the child's health and safety is paramount.

A Social Worker Responds

Because she was convicted of attempting to murder Nat, Rose's parental rights would almost certainly have been terminated even though Nat is living with a relative. As a result, Nat would either be in the permanent custody of Rose's aunt or would have been adopted by her. If a suitable kinship placement had not been available Nat would have been placed in the home of a foster family that was qualified and willing to adopt him. For reasons stated above, the fate of Rose's unborn child would follow a similar path—he/she would be placed in protective custody upon birth and the mother's parental rights terminated. The infant would be placed in either kinship care, ideally with the aunt who is caring for Nat, or in an adoption-eligible foster home.

Given this scenario, it is unlikely that the state would permit Rose to have visits with her children during and following her incarceration unless the state believed it was in the best interests of the children and it could convince the court of jurisdiction that such was the case; this would be very difficult to accomplish.

Research has found that 92 per cent of the children of incarcerated mothers experience some kind of severe or chronic problem. The most common mental health challenges include separation anxiety, depression, and aggressive behavior. Many of these children have significant physical health problems. Consequently, the social worker in this case should ensure that Nat receives services to ameliorate or prevent these problems. These services would include mental health therapy, academic tracking and support, and medical services. Research has also demonstrated that these children experience highly unstable living situations and often experience multiple separations from caregivers, the consequences of which are manifest in the problems described above. In light of these findings, the social worker involved in this case would provide services designed to support the development and stability of the relationship between Nat and his mother's aunt and other family members (Dally, 2002; Poehlmann, 2005).

Children of incarcerated parents face many negative life challenges that lead to negative self-evaluation, social stigma, and isolation. These act as barriers to accessing resources that help them feel less marginalized. Moreover, children of an incarcerated parent sometimes lack role models, especially since the incarcerated parent is not a person in whose footsteps the child can follow. Consequently, they need resources such as support groups, mentoring, and other kinds of social support (Nesmith, Ruhland & Krueger, 2006).

The social worker in this case should work with Nat's caregiver to create a plan for regularly sharing information about his mother's condition and living situation. If the state and court deem it to be in Nat's best interest to have contact with his mother, then the social worker would ensure that this contact occurs through mail, electronic communication, phone, or in person. Most children prefer to visit and spend time with their incarcerated parent and this dramatically increases the chances of reunification.

Nevertheless, significant barriers to successful visitation exist including distance to facilities, uncomfortable and unaccommodating visiting rooms, and inflexible visitation regulations (Davis, Landsverk, Newton, & Ganger, 1996). If Nat were permitted to visit his mother, the social worker should provide or arrange for transportation to and from the facility and ensure that the visits are as comfortable as possible for the child.

Studies of incarcerated mothers who were living with their children prior to their incarceration report that most have few job skills, lack educational qualifications, and struggle to support themselves and their children. Most of these women come from difficult family backgrounds involving incarceration, drug abuse, and physical and sexual abuse. In addition, many of these women were involved with the juvenile justice and child welfare systems as children. Most have significant substance abuse histories (Dalley, 2002; Greene, Haney, & Hurtado, 2000). Almost 80 per cent of the women in the Dalley study reported that they had been "habitual" drug users and that their addiction interfered with their relationships with and ability to care for their children. Moreover, many of these women are developmentally delayed and lack the ability for abstract thinking and understanding cause-and-effect relationships. Given these findings, the social worker assigned to help Rose would need to assess the degree to which these issues have impacted her in the past and create a plan for minimizing the impacts in the future.

Services might include substance abuse treatment, individual and group therapy focusing on trauma resolution and loss and grief resulting from separation from Nat, and the development of insight. Rose would likely benefit from parenting classes which are offered at most correctional facilities (Hoffman, Byrd, & Knighlinger, 2010). The social worker would also work to help Rose obtain her high school diploma and additional post-secondary education to increase her ability to secure lawful and gainful employment.

Although it is highly unlikely in this case, if Rose were permitted to retain parental rights and have contact with her newborn child, the social worker would work to help her spend as much time as possible with the infant. According to Byrne, Goshin, and Joestl (2010), infants who live with their incarcerated mothers in a prison nursery for more than one year are significantly more likely to become securely attached to their mother regardless of the quality of the mother's attachment representation. Other programs such as "Girl Scouts Beyond Bars: Facilitating Parent-Child Contact in Correctional Settings" assist incarcerated parents in bonding with their children for the first time, or preserving or fortifying the bond interrupted by incarceration (Block & Potthast, 1998). The social worker should help Rose access these types of resources if available.

Regardless of whether or not Rose is allowed to have contact with her children she should be updated regarding their development and well-being (Nesmith et al., 2006). Therefore, the social worker should facilitate a connection between Rose and her children even if contact is not possible.

Exercises

In class

The following exercises are for class discussion and debate and might elicit different responses from members of the groups. A respectful and supportive atmosphere should be maintained at all times regardless of the varying dimensions of individual viewpoints.

- If you were a social worker involved in any one of the foregoing cases, how would you respond? In what way and why would your response be different from those presented in this chapter?

- What are the cultural parameters regarding different types of family conflict in your society and how do social workers manage such situations?
- Do international protocols provide any consistent guidance in dealing with family conflict in a variety of settings?

Outside of class

For each of the exercises below select a country different from your home country and those discussed in this chapter. Present your findings to your peers in class on the following:

- Gather information on another country that describes and debates family conflict on a variety of issues and summarized related concerns and challenges.
- Consider the legal aspects of concerns related to conflict in the family and compare and contrast them to those in your home country.
- Conduct a comparative literature review of two countries and their approach to different aspects of family conflict highlighting how social workers in both might perceive and utilize this information.
- Develop a list of agencies in your country that work with conflictual family relationships and make suggestions for addressing any gaps in their response to such issues.
- Obtain the views of two social workers in your community on specific issues related to family conflict and the community's formal and informal response thereto.

References

Adoption and Safe Families Act (1997). Retrieved from http://www.acf.hhs.gov/programs/cb/laws_policies/cblaws/public_law/p1105_89.htm

Block, K., & Potthast, M. (1998). Girl scouts beyond bars: Facilitating parent-child contact in a correctional setting. *Child Welfare*, 77 (5), 561–78.

Byrne, M., Goshin, L., & Joestl, S. (2010). Intergenerational transmission of attachment for infants raised in a prison nursery. *Attachment & Human Development*, 12 (4), 375–93

Child Care Act (1991). "Care Proceedings." Retrieved from <www.irishstatutebook.ie/1991/en/act/pub/0017/index.html>

Citterio, E. (2010). "Untapped skills: Refugees and labor market in South Africa." Retrieved from www.afronline.org

Canadian Bar Association (CBA) (2010). "Common-law relationships: What happens when your spouse dies." Retrieved from http://www.cba.org/bc/public_media/family/150.aspx

Canadian Cancer Society (2011). "General cancer statistics at a glance." Retrieved from http://www.cancer.ca/Canadaide/About%20cancer/Cancer%20statistics/Stats%20at%20a%20glance/General%20cancer%20stats.aspx?sc_lang=en#ixzz1TQxdWoZA

Canadian Association of Social Workers (CASW). (2008) "CASW scope of practice statement." Retrieved from http://www.casw-acts.ca/sites/default/files/attachements/Scope%20of%20Practice_August_08_E_Final.pdf

Dalley, L. P., (2002). "Policy implications relating to inmate mothers and their children: Will the past be prologue?" *The Prison Journal, 82* (2), 234–68.

Davis, I. P., Landsverk, J., Newton, R., & Ganger, W. (1996). "Parental visiting and foster care reunification." *Children and Youth Services Review,* 18 (4/5), 363–82.

Germain, C. B., & Gitterman, A. (1996). *The life model of social work practice.* (2nd edn). New York Columbia University Press.

Government of Alberta (2005). "Responding to child abuse: A handbook." Retrieved from: http://www.solgps.alberta.ca/safe_communities/community_awareness/family_violence/Publications/Responding%20to%20child%20abuse%20handbook.pdf

Government of British Columbia (2007). "The BC handbook for action on child abuse and neglect." Retrieved from www.bced.gov.bc.ca/sco/resourcedocs/handbook_action_child_abuse.pdf

Government of Saskatchewan (2010). "Saskatchewan child welfare review panel report: For the good of our children and youth." Retrieved from: http://www.bced.gov.bc.ca/sco/resourcedocs/handbook_action_child_abuse.pdf

Greene, S., Haney, C., & Hurtado, A. (2000). "Cycles of pain: Risk factors in the lives of incarcerated mothers and their children." *The Prison Journal,* 80 (1), 3–23.

Hariston, C. F. (2004). "Prisoners and families: Parenting issues during incarceration." In J. Travis & M. Waul (Eds.). *Prisoners and families: Parenting issues during incarceration* (pp. 259–84). Washington, D.C.: The Urban Press Institute.

Hoffman, H. C., Byrd, A. L., & Knighlinger, A. M. (2010). "Prison programs and services for incarcerated parents and their underage children: Results from a national survey of correctional facilities." *The Prison Journal,* 90 (4), 397–416.

Human Resources and Skill Development Canada (HRSDC) (2000). "Child welfare in Canada 2000." Retrieved from http://www.hrsdc.gc.ca/eng/cs/sp/sdc/socpol/publications/reports/2000-000033/page03.shtml

IndexMundi (2011a). "Canada – Demographics profile 2011." Retrieved from http://www.indexmundi.com/canada/demographics_profile.html

Indian Evidence Act, (1972). Retrieved from http://www.vakilno1.com/bareacts/indianevidenceact/indicanevidenceact.htm

Lamanna, M. A., & Riedmann, A. C. (2006). *Marriages & families: Making choices and facing change.* (9th edn). Belmont, CA: Thomson/Wadsworth.

Manicom, C. (2010). "Psychosocial cancer care." *Continuing Medical Education (CME)*. 28 (2): 58–63

Mauer, M., Nellis, A., & Schirmer, S. (2007). "Incarcerated parents and their children-Trends 1991–2007." Retrieved from www.sentencingproject.org

Mulcahy, M., & Trocme, N. (2010). "Children and youth in out-of-home care in Canada." CECW Information Sheet #78E. Retrieved from http://www.cecwcepb.ca/sites/default/files/publications/en/ChildrenInCare78E.pdf

National Resource Center on Children and Families of the Incarcerated (2011). "Report." Retrieved from http://fcnetwork.org/resources/fact-sheets

Nesmith, A., Ruhland, E., & Krueger, S. (2006). "Children of incarcerated parents." *Council on Crime and Justice*. Retrieved from http://www.gcyf.org/usr_doc/CCJ_CIP_Final_Report.pdf http://sfreentry.com/wp-content/uploads/2010/01/2010-01-28-bib-FVC-cms-nwb1.pdf

Ottawa Citizen (2007). "Canadians want illegal immigrants deported: Poll." Retrieved from http://www.canada.com/nationalpost/news/story.html?id=f86690ed-a2ed-447c-8be8-21ba5a3dd922

Poehlmann, J. (2005). "Representations of attachment relationships in children of incarcerated mothers." *Child Development*, 76 (3), 679–696.

Public Health Agency of Canada (2009). "HIV and AIDS surveillance report." Retrieved from http://www.phac-aspc.gc.ca/aids-sida/publication/survreport/2009/dec/index-eng.php. Refugee Act 1998. South Africa. No. 130.

Weigel, D. J. (2008). "The concept of family: An analysis of laypeople's views of family." *Journal of Family Issues*, 29 (11), 1426–47.

Weiser, S. D., Leiter, K., Heisler, M., et al. (2006). "A population-based study on alcohol and high risk sexual behaviours in Botswana." *PLoS Medicine*, 3 (10), 1940–47.

Wilson, A. (1985). *Family*. London: Routledge.

World Health Organization (WHO) (2008). Retrieved from http://www.who.int/mental-health/prevention/suicide/suiciderates/en/

6 Elder Care/ Elder Populations

By Caren J. Frost

Socio-demographic patterns in the aging population continue to change with statistics showing an increasing rate of aging people at 2.6 per cent annually (UN, 2010). With improved medical care and health services, life expectancy rates continue to improve in most countries. However, this trend presents societies with new challenges, particularly in areas such as caring for the aged. In the cultural context of individualist and collectivist societies, there are both positive and negative views of the elderly. Such views indicate that in some cultural constructs the elderly may generally be viewed as being genial, while in other cultural views the elderly may be viewed as being ineffectual and lacking in certain capacities (Cuddy, Norton & Fiske, 2005).

Elderly populations are more prominent to certain disorders and conditions (Feldman & Damron-Rodriguez, 2007; Lamanna & Riedmann, 2006; UN, n.d.; Davies & Higginson, 2004). Nevertheless, the family remains an important informal agent in providing care for the elderly. As is illustrated in this chapter, the dynamics of the relationship between parents and children may influence the nature of care given to aging parents (Lamanna & Riedmann, 2006). This interplay can create tensions and be a precipitating factor for elder abuse. Research indicates that there is a correlation between the quality of the social relations and interactions elderly people have and their well-being (Antonucci, Okorodudu & Akiyama, 2002). Thus maintaining family connections and social support in their known communities is important to the elderly. Another aspect of aging in that grandparents in many families provide assistance with childcare when primary caregivers or family instability seems to be a concern. This chapter will present information about all of these issues.

Family Caregiving for the Elderly

BY MARILYN LUPTAK FROM THE US

Jane Olson is an 82-year-old female who was diagnosed with Alzheimer's disease—the most common type of dementia—four years ago. Her other health problems include high blood pressure, mild chronic obstructive pulmonary disease, and slight hearing loss. She lives with Douglas Olson, her 83-year-old husband of many years, in their two-storey home in a working-class neighborhood of a metropolitan area. John, their oldest son (age 60), lives 90 miles away and tries to visit them every two to three months. Their other children, Martin (age 55) and Nancy (age 58), live in other parts of the country and rarely come home to visit.

Mrs Olson's most recent mental examination score is 16/30, which means she is in the moderate stage of Alzheimer's disease. She is able to transfer and ambulate with cueing and assistance. She also needs help taking her medications, bathing, dressing, using the bathroom, eating, and other daily activities.

Mr Olson, who has rheumatoid arthritis, provides supervision and help 24 hours a day, seven days a week—assisting his wife with daily activities and getting up with her at night. He is proud that he has not used any formal community services such as care coordination, counseling, activity and support groups, home health care and adult day center programs. However, Mrs Olson has recently developed some problems with swallowing and it is increasingly difficult for him to feed her. It now takes him one and a half hours to feed her at mealtimes and he is finding it hard to keep up with managing their finances, shopping, laundry, meal preparation, and other household chores. As a result, he is physically exhausted, experiencing high levels of emotional stress, and has started to consider placing Mrs Olson in a nursing home.

Family Caregiving for the Elderly: A Social Worker from the US Responds

BY JENNIFER HUGHES

Prevalence and Incidence

According to "Caregiving in the US," a study conducted by the National Alliance for Caregiving (2009), an estimated 65.7 million people have served as unpaid family caregivers to an adult or a child in the past 12 months. These caregivers are predominately female (66 per cent) with an average age of 48 years. The vast majority of caregivers provide care for a relative (86 per cent) with over one-third taking care of a parent (36 per cent). In this study, caregivers were asked the main reason their recipient needed care; the top two issues they reported were old age (12 per cent) and Alzheimer's disease or dementia (10 per cent). Other care needs were mental/emotional illness (7 per cent), cancer (7 per cent), heart disease (5 per cent), and stroke (5 per cent). On average, caregivers spend 20.4 hours per week providing care (Caregiving in the US, 2009).

Country Policies

The US Department of Human Services Administration in Aging offers the National Family Caregiver Support Program (NFCSP) (2000) under Title IIIE of the Older Americans Act of 1965, which is specifically targeted to provide caregiver assistance. This program provides assistance for caregivers to keep family members at home for as long as possible. With this program, families are able to receive counseling, group support, training, respite care, and information and referral services. This program was designed to work in conjunction with other state and community services and provide a coordinated set of support services with an effort to reduce the cost of institutional or long-term care (Administration on Aging 2011).

A Social Worker Responds

A social worker in the US might respond to this case by providing a coordination of care services approach. The social worker would link available services focused on addressing the needs of both the informal caregiver and care receiver with specific attention to helping both care partners enjoy an improved quality of life. The social worker would consider service eligibility, service availability, and financial reimbursement along with the provision of quality care when developing a case plan for this care system.

The worker would begin by concerning him/herself with the client's and caregiver's right to self-determination, and seek client and care provider input for decision making regarding case outcome. Assurance of client confidentiality and ethical decision making considerations are also important issues for the social worker. It is important for the social worker to understand that the husband caregiver expressed satisfaction and pride over his ability to care for his wife without formal community assistance. The social worker would educate the caregiver from a disease perspective, and help him become comfortable with the idea of using services to assist him in the care of his wife while developing an understanding that his wife's illness will become progressively worse.

In this particular case, the care receiver is experiencing a moderate stage of Alzheimer's disease, and she will begin to require extensive assistance including round the clock care, bathing, dressing, feeding, personal need assistance, and protection from the environment. The social worker should introduce the concept of long-term care options to the caregiver and begin to suggest gradual amounts of care assistance while bearing in mind the caregiver's potential resistance to out-of-home help. With time and understanding, the caregiver may see the benefit of utilizing such service programs and realize that long-term care options will allow his wife to remain as independent as possible for as long as possible. Long-term care programs in the US can include home health care, case management, transportation, escort services, homemaker services, night sitting, recreation, nursing home care, adult day care, personal care attendants, and home meals. Additionally, specialized care for individuals with cognitive and functional impairments is available in situations involving Alzheimer's and dementia.

A social worker specializing in elderly care would understand that the caregiver will undoubtedly feel overwhelmed if too many options or services were instituted at once. The social worker should assess the client from a strength-based case management perspective and provide the opportunity to introduce services as needed while planning ahead and providing future long-term care options. The emphasis for this client system is on the quality of life and the quality of care for both client and care provider while understanding the gradual loss that will occur during this disease process.

Involvement of extended family members to ensure choice and quality of care should additionally be considered in this case even though the adult children live at a distance. Case planning support from adult children may help both the care receiver and caregiver through the transition to more formal care assistance. The adult children may help their parents understand the need and importance of assistance and even encourage the parents to comfortably utilize long-term care services.

Throughout the social worker's involvement with this family, the continuum of care or least restricted care environment becomes an important consideration. It is essential that the care receiver remain in the least restrictive environment possible. Change and movement to more restricted care surroundings will occur as abilities diminish; however, providing support and encouragement for aging and disabled populations to live in the least restrictive environment as long as possible is essential to social work practice. It is important to convey this treatment goal to the caregiver early so that Mr Olson becomes comfortable with the treatment plan and goals and does not feel powerless. If the care provider understands that keeping the care receiver in the home with assistance as long as possible is the treatment goal, the caregiver may feel more comfortable allowing care assistance in his home.

There are additional considerations regarding this case which include some legal aspects, care availability, and financial reimbursement. From a legal perspective, advanced directives should be discussed with the care receiver, care provider, and their adult children. Plans for future care and long-term health decisions can be extremely useful in addressing end-of-life care. Providing an opportunity for discussion to facilitate advanced directives will be helpful. Another consideration for this case is access and availability to care options. Available services for the family will significantly direct the treatment plan. Not all services are available in all areas, and services available in a rural versus urban setting may differ. Typically, more varied options are available in more urban areas. For instance, services like adult day care or "meals on wheels" (a food delivery program) may not be available in a rural area. Finally, financial resources are important in developing a care plan. In the US, Medicaid is a primary financial support for long-term care. The social worker will need to check on the available reimbursement options for the couple and potentially help the care provider apply for Medicaid or Medicare, if necessary. The couple may have access to supplemental or managed care health insurance, which might assist in providing financial assistance for long-term care options. The social worker might need to advocate for the client system with the potential financiers to secure coverage for the client. The client system may have personal funds to help cover the high costs of care options. Financial considerations will also direct the care plan because not all clients will have access to needed health care coverage.

In summary, providing social work services for a family caregiving situation with the elderly must consider both the care receiver's and care provider's needs and abilities. With respect to the client's right to self-determination, maintaining the client in the least restrictive environment as long as possible is an important consideration when caring for patients with Alzheimer's disease. A variety of long-term care options are available in the US and social workers can facilitate services to the client system. It is also important for the social worker to work closely with the care provider and value the caregiver and the extended family members' dignity and decision making ability in this situation as well.

Family Caregiving for the Elderly: A Social Worker from South Korea Responds

BY HYUN SOOK KIM, YONG-JUNG KWON, & HANNAH NAM (ENGLISH TRANSLATION)

Prevalence and Incidence

Social security expenses for people aged 65 and over are increasing rapidly. As of 2009, national pension recipients aged 65 and over consisted 27.6 per cent of total recipients, which is an 11.5 per cent increase since 2005 (16.1 per cent). In 2009, national health insurance paid the health care service costs of 12.0391 trillion Korean Won for people aged 65 and over, which accounts for 30.5 per cent of total health care service costs.

The most difficult problems that the Korean elderly population faces are reported as "economic difficulties (41.4 per cent)" and "health problems (40.3 per cent)" (Ministry of Health and Welfare, 2009). Based on a study of community elderly populations (65 years of age and above) in 2008 (Ministry of Health and Welfare, 2009), 84.9 per cent of the population had at least one physician-diagnosed disease. The disease prevalence in descending order was hypertension (44.4 per cent), osteoarthritis/rheumatoid arthritis (27.4 per cent), back pain/sciatica (17.0 per cent), diabetes mellitus (15.6 per cent), and osteoporosis (12.4 per cent). At least 82 per cent of elderly persons reported that the diseases had an impact on their daily lives with extreme difficulty reported by 30.1 per cent and slight difficulty reported by 51.9 per cent. Additionally, 30.8 per cent of the elderly reported some degree of depression.

South Korea is a rapidly evolving society with increasing economic problems for the elderly and weakening of familial bonds. Thus, depression and suicide among the elderly has become an emerging issue. As of 2009, 4,071 deaths in the population of 65 years and above can be attributed to suicide.

The rapidly aging society has also contributed to the increase in the number of people with dementia. Several population studies estimate the prevalence of seniors living with dementia at between 6.3 per cent and 13 per cent; as of 2008, the number of patients 65 and above suffering from dementia was estimated to be about 420,000, or about 8.2 per cent of the population. If the number of patients with dementia continues to expand at this rate, it is extrapolated that there will be about half a million dementia patients by 2012, 1 million by 2027, and 2.12 million by 2050. In 2008, the most prevalent types of dementia were Alzheimer's (71 per cent), vascular dementia (24 per cent), and other types (5 per cent).

Country Policies

South Korea has developed a variety of health insurance and aid programs for short-term and long-term care with each having its own qualification criteria as well as costs and intervention strategies. The National Health Insurance Program is compulsory social insurance, which covers the entire native Korean population residing in the country. Major sources financing this program are contributions from the insured and government subsidies.

The Medical Aid Program is the government's medical benefit program, and is a form of public assistance to secure the minimum livelihood of low-income households and assist with self-help by providing medical services. The Long-Term Care Insurance Program began in July 2008 when the Korean government introduced long-term care insurance to ease the financial burden on family caregivers with no income. It was designed to satisfy the needs of Korean senior citizens who have difficulty performing their daily activities due to geriatric diseases.

In-home services available for the elderly include visitor home care, visitor bathing, skilled nursing care, day and night care, and short-term respite care. Other types of care, such as the rental service of welfare equipment (manual wheelchair, ambulatory bathtub, in-tub bath lift or anti-bedsore mattress) are also available at a low cost to beneficiaries who stay out of long-term care facilities. Long-term care facility services provide all services residents require except groceries, medical equipment, haircuts and beauty products, and extra fees for patients to upgrade their hospital rooms. Long-term care insurance services also provide special cash benefits, for example family care cash benefits, exceptional care cash benefits, and nursing expenses of long-term care hospitals.

The approval process for long-term care benefits involves the following steps through which clients, caregivers, and/or social workers negotiate:

1 Applying for long-term care benefits;
2 Completing an examination for approval by National Health Insurance Cooperation;
3 Submitting a medical opinion by a client;
4 Completing an assessment and obtaining an assigned rate by referring to written examination, medical opinion, and other documents by the Need Assessment Committee;
5 Sending in the long-term care approval certificate and standardized long-term care utilization plan;
6 Creating a long-term care benefits contract followed by using the benefits by beneficiaries and long-term care institutions.

A Social Worker Responds

In South Korea, this case would normally be managed by social workers using a case management approach. The process of assessment—plan—intervention—monitoring—evaluation—reassessment would be applied. Thus the first step for a social worker would be to review and assess the client (Mrs Olson) and her family caregiver from various angles. The social worker would try to identify exactly what Mr Olson's needs are. The initial focus would be to assist Mr Olson in expressing how he wants the details of his wife's disease and resulting difficulties to be managed.

The social worker would conduct an assessment of both Mrs Olson and her husband. See Table 1 for an example.

The Olson's resources would be assessed. Their formal resources would be categorized as unknown and their informal resources would be noted as their three adult children. From this information, strengths for this couple would be considered. For example, their oldest son, John who is a 60-year-old male, is interested in the care of his parents, which is a good resource for the Olsons. It is clear that Mr Olson is able to assist his wife in certain activities of daily living. Due to Mrs Olson's physical and mental health issues (moderate dementia, hypertension, mild COPD, hearing loss) as well as her impairments (ADL & IADL—difficulties with swallowing), some services will need to be identified and made available to the couple if Mr Olson wants to keep his wife in their home. Thus the intervention plans for each of these problems are considered in terms of health care and social services. This case will require an integrated approach between both health care and social services; the primary intervention plan would involve Mrs Olson's deteriorating ability to function, as these difficulties in her caregiving are the main reason behind the mental and physical stress that Mr Olson is experiencing.

Table 1 Assessment of Mrs and Mr Olson's Needs and/or Problems

Problem or Need	Assessment	
	Client Jane Olson (82 year old female)	**Primary Caregiver** Douglas Olson (83 year old male)
Physical Health	– Diagnosed with moderate Alzheimer's disease 4 years ago, MMSE score 16/30 – Hypertension, mild COPD, slight hearing loss	– Rheumatoid arthritis – 24/7 caregiving activities for significant other – Extreme physical fatigue due to caregiving activities
Mental Health		– High levels of emotional stress due to caregiving activities – Proud that he has not found need to utilize formal community services
ADL & IADL	– Needs help taking her medications, bathing, dressing, using the bathroom, eating, and other daily activities	– Difficulty assisting significant other in eating – Difficulties with managing finances, shopping, laundry, meal preparation, and other household chores
Others		– Considering placement of significant other in nursing home

A secondary intervention plan involving Mr Olson can be established after progress with Mrs Olson is adequately monitored. The establishment of rapport with the couple through healthy and honest communication, including a thorough discussion of available options with Mr Olson, will be vital in achieving these end goals, especially since Mr Olson seems somewhat averse to utilizing formal community services and is proud that he has not needed them until now. Mr Olson's wishes would be fully considered in establishing a care plan for any interventions.

With the permission of Mr Olson, the Olsons would apply for long-term care benefits from the National Health Insurance Corporation. If approval for the long-term care benefits is classified as rating 1–3, the following plan can be established. If the approval is less than a level 3, it is possible to refer the Olsons to an out-of-pocket nursing service depending on their finances or to an in-home service provided by the local district or community. In the latter case, each facility will have a designated social worker to provide case management. The social worker will most likely be employed by

Table 2 Short-term Care Plan

Priority	Goals	Service Planning			
		Service form	Provider	Time Period or Frequency	Fee
1	Allow client to function in ADL with assistance Decrease caregiver stress	Counseling service	Social welfare centers for the elderly	PRN	Free
		Visiting home care service	Long-term care facility	Every day, 4 hours per day	Out of pocket (15%)
		Visiting bath	Long-term care facility	2x per week	Out of pocket (15%)
		Management of elderly with dementia	Community health center	1x per month	Free
		Support groups for families with dementia	Social welfare center for the elderly	1x per week	Free
2	Maintain current health with medication management	Community health service (door-to-door)	Community health center	1x per week	Free

the Community Welfare Center. The activities from the short-term plan indicate the time and frequency of visiting services, as well as personal hygiene maintenance services which can be adjusted based on Mrs Olson's needs. The fee for services not covered by national health insurance and co-payment of health insurance (5 per cent–20 per cent) would probably be provided by the Olson's oldest son unless the Olson's can afford it.

In terms of a long-term care plan, Mrs Olson is experiencing significant functional difficulties, and Mr Olson has health issues that make living in a two-storey house increasingly difficult. One option might be to provide information on moving to a smaller, single-storey house requiring less maneuvering and utilizing the remaining finances from selling their larger house to supplement payment for increased visiting services. A second option would be to refer the clients to a long-term care facility if they so desired.

If Mrs Olson is approved for a long-term care benefit, Mr Olson should explore utilizing community social welfare centers for the elderly and possibly have more personal time to socialize with peers and enjoy different cultural activities. This benefit will allow Mr Olson to separate himself from the immediate stress of caregiving, de-stress, and establish a new relationship with his wife in terms of caregiving. Although the time Mr Olson spends with his wife may lessen, sound mental health will lead to an increase in the quality of the time he spends with her. Another important activity would be to have the Olsons reconnect and bond with their children through more frequent communication. Education in the utilization of new technology such as video conferences will help achieve these goals. The social worker would provide continuous monitoring (every 30 days) to determine how the Olsons are responding to the services and plans. In this way there would be assurance that their needs are being met through the identified interventions.

Case study #2

Grandparents Caring for Grandchildren because Parents are Absent

BY TSHEPO MOGAPI FROM BOTSWANA

Sam, a 69-year-old grandfather, is raising his 11-year-old HIV-positive granddaughter, Ruth. They reside in a small village. In 1999, just after she was born, Ruth came to live with her grandfather. At that time, she was very sick and her mother had just passed away from AIDS. Sam realized then that Ruth was HIV positive. He was distressed with the results since he did not know how the child acquired the virus. He does not know a lot about HIV and AIDS. He said he only knew that HIV starts like tuberculosis and then the person will eventually become very sick.

Sam is unemployed and it is difficult for him to put food on the table. At times, Sam is not able to attend social gatherings or funerals due to Ruth's frequent illnesses and hospitalizations. However, he believes that it is his responsibility to care for his granddaughter.

During the recent school holidays, Sam and Ruth went to the cattle post, where the family keeps their livestock. However, Ruth had to leave early to return to their village for an appointment. She was accompanied by her cousin, Carol, who was the same age as Ruth (11). On their way to their village, the children were given a ride by a male stranger. Just as they approached the village, Ruth was sexually assaulted and then raped by this man. Ruth told Sam about the incident two days later when he arrived from the cattle post. He reported the case to the police and Ruth was treated at the local hospital.

At this time, Ruth was showing signs of emotional disturbance: she was withdrawn and not playing with other children. She only felt safe around her grandfather. Sam felt guilty about the rape since he felt that if he had been there he could have prevented it from happening. Carol, Ruth's cousin, is also hurting and continually weeps and sobs with her cousin.

Ruth seems to be experiencing an emotional upheaval. She is self conscious about almost everything around her including the way people look at her, what people say, and how her family members treat her. It seems that nobody is in a position to answer the many questions she wants to ask them. These are questions such as: Why me? How could this man be so cruel to choose me when there were two of us? Why am I suffering like this? Although the family tries to be supportive in every possible way, it is obvious that they too have been deeply affected by the incident. The family is angry and frustrated, and feels that its burden has been doubled. First, they had Ruth's HIV to deal with and now they have to help her deal with the rape which will change her life forever. The repercussions are enormous and tension seems to mount with every passing day. At this point, the hospital staff encourages the family to consult the hospital social worker for support.

Grandparents Caring for Grandchildren because Parents are Absent: A Social Worker from the US Responds

BY TROY CHRISTIAN ANDERSON

Prevalence and Incidence

According to the US Census Bureau there were 6.2 million children under age 18 residing with a grandparent in 2007; of this number, 2.6 million relied on the grandparent for primary care provision (US Census 2007). This total accounts for 9 per cent of all children in the US Poverty and ethnic diversity are key risk factors in increased rates of kinship care. The need for grandparents to assume a primary care role is more common in African

American communities, affecting approximately 12 per cent of children in this ethnic group compared to 7 per cent of Hispanic households and 4 per cent of non-Hispanic white children (Baker, Silverstein, & Putney, 2008).

Country Policies

There has been a lack of recognition of kinship care as a formal and lasting social construct, which has led to delays in formal policies aimed at assisting grandparents in caring for their grandchildren. In 2000, the National Family Caregiver Support Program was enacted as a component of the Older Americans Act. Ten per cent of funding from this program is allocated for grandparents who are over age 60. Services offered include resource referrals, family counseling, support groups, and respite services (Lent, 2005). In addition, there have been policy changes targeted at supporting grandparents in their primary care provision role. One example is changes in the laws that determine access to medical and educational decision making for kinship care providers who do not have a formal legal relationship. This change is occurring on a state-by-state basis. Finally, an ongoing barrier that impacts the most vulnerable of care providers is limited access to financial assistance through public aid programs. Grandparents have been found to be less likely to access these programs even when a clear need exists (Goodman, Potts, & Pasztor, 2007).

A Social Worker Responds

This case poses a real-life scenario that challenges even a seasoned clinical social worker. To address the multilevel needs of this family in crisis, a clinical social worker is required to possess clinical and diagnostic acumen, community resource expertise on both a local and national level, and crisis intervention skills. The outlined steps will proceed in perceived urgency with critical needs addressed first.

Ruth is in immediate need of emergency medical and mental health interventions. After her immediate medical needs are addressed in the local emergency room, Ruth requires an emergency appointment at the infectious disease out-patient clinic at a local University Health Science Center. It is critical that her HIV status be measured immediately to determine if she could have possibly been reinfected with the HI virus or other sexually transmitted diseases as a result of her rape. While there, she and her grandfather will be referred to the clinical social worker in order to fully educate them about the causes, complications, lifestyle considerations, and prevention of complications of the HI virus. Finally, it is critical that Ruth continues to develop an age appropriate understanding of HIV. Sessions with the infectious disease social worker would be scheduled and continue until the social worker feels that Ruth has a well-developed understanding of how best to care for herself and her chronic disease.

Immediately after the medical appointment, Ruth will be referred to the local Rape Crisis Center for immediate mental health treatment. Trauma induced by a rape, especially at a young age, requires immediate attention to mediate the severity of the effects of the trauma. In conjunction with her treatment, it will also be necessary that her grandfather receive education regarding the effects of trauma, as well as common symptoms and warning signs related to this type of event. Finally, seeking intervention at this facility would also be beneficial for Carol because she witnessed the traumatic event and also needs immediate assistance. Funding for the services available at the Rape Crisis Center would be sought through Crime Victims Reparation, a resource dedicated to support the medical and mental health needs of individuals impacted by violent crime.

Once the immediate crises have been addressed, it is critical to assess the secondary needs of the family, who lack the financial resources to provide for even their most basic needs. Ruth is eligible for Utah's CHIP (Children's Health Insurance Program) and TANF (Temporary Assistance for Needy Families) to assist with basic financial sustenance. Sam is eligible for Medicare and Medicaid due to his financial difficulties. Application for all of the entitlement programs would be initiated immediately; and through the evaluation a determination would be made about all the programs that are available to help financially support this family unit. Finally, Social Security would be contacted to determine if Ruth is eligible for a survivor benefit due to her mother's death. If so, appropriate applications would be completed.

In addition to the therapy set up specifically to address the rape-related issues, it is important that Ruth and Sam have ongoing out-patient mental health follow-up and support. Initiating the next level of care could wait until the treatment is resolved at the Rape Crisis Center. The focus of this intervention would address issues with ongoing support and adjustment to the family's unique situation. Resources would be available to cover the costs of the intervention once Medicaid and CHIP insurance funding is established.

To further support his role as a grandparent raising a grandchild, Sam would be referred to an agency with a primary mission to support older individuals involved with kinship care. The Children's Service Society provides support with seeking financial help and other general support services to grandparents. They offer a 12-week class on the basics of kinship care. Programs are also available that offer holiday events for grandparents and their grandchildren. Finally, support groups exist for the children and these meet at the same time as older adult groups.

It is critical that a plan addresses the issue of adding longer term support for Sam's role as a primary care provider for Ruth. An appointment would be established to assess Sam's social support system. This support is important on at least two levels. First, Sam needs support in his current role as a primary parent. The preventive and proactive use of respite (scheduled breaks from the caregiving role) is vital to allow Sam to continue in this role as long as possible. Research indicates that care providers are likely to suffer poor mental and physical health. It is likely that Sam will not live long enough to see Ruth into adulthood. A well established plan will address both short-term and permanent plans for support in case of changes in his care provision abilities. The first circle of potential support is Sam's immediate and extended family system. Careful exploration will seek to identify anyone that can play a role in providing preventive respite support and possible back-up care of Ruth.

The next level of assistance to be explored is extended potential community support beyond the family circle. The discussion would include neighbors, church, community, and other structured lay support. Once this circle has been exhausted, contacts with community and professional programs would be explored. An ideal respite system would include structured and predictable breaks for Sam. Setting up a "call when I need help" approach should be avoided. It is the structured and scheduled nature of the respite support that actually provides the preventive aspects of respite. If the only time Sam gets a break coincides with scheduled appointments or other necessary demands, Sam is not getting the reprieve he needs. This structured respite program should allow Sam to have free and unstructured time to pursue other activities that he enjoys.

Finally, the family would require ongoing periodic monitoring of their situation. This task could be accomplished by either their ongoing out-patient mental health counselor or a social worker who is engaged in a case management role. Infrequent updates could manage new concerns that arise and unexpected situations could be addressed on an urgent basis. Due to the complex nature of the interventions required, it would be beneficial to have a case manager who is familiar with the various services utilize.

Grandparents Caring for Grandchildren because Parents are Absent: A Social Worker from Finland Responds

BY JUHA HÄMÄLÄINEN, RIITTA VORNANEN, PIRJO PÖLKKI, & LEENA LEINONEN

Prevalence and Incidence

According to a UN study on violence against children (2006), girls are at a greater risk of sexual violence than boys. In Finland, the majority of sexually abused children are girls. According to a recent study by Laaksonen, et al., (2011), the prevalence of child sexual abuse (CSA) has declined in Finland during the last two decades in comparison with earlier studies by Sariola and Uutela (1994; 1996). A simultaneous decline has occurred in factors associated with CSA.

The data in the aforementioned study were based on the responses of 4,561 men (Mean age = 29, Standard Deviation = seven years) and 8,361 females (Mean age = 29, Standard Deviation = seven years) to the Childhood Trauma Questionnaire (Short Form), as well as to questions regarding family structure. The prevalence of CSA experiences varied between 0.7 per cent and 4.6 per cent for men, and 1.8 per cent and 7.5 per cent for women, depending on the item involved. Younger cohorts reported fewer instances of CSA, as well as fewer risk factors that were positively associated with the likelihood of CSA (physical neglect and abuse, emotional neglect and abuse, parental substance abuse, not growing up with both biological parents). The effects of the risk factors did not vary as a function of cohort. The declining trend was not explainable by higher social desirability among the younger cohorts.

Antikainen (2005) reviewed published studies to profile the risks of children's sexual abuse. In Finland, a higher percentage of sexually-abused children are from foreign backgrounds. Children with mental disabilities or psychological or physical differences also may be at increased risk of sexual abuse. Sexually-abused children more often lived in single-parent, low income households, and less frequently lived with both of their biological parents (Antikainen, 2005). Parental loss or separation often heightens vulnerability (see also Waterston & Mok, 2008), which is evaluated from a social work perspective in this analysis.

Country Policies

After World War II, and especially in the period after 1960, the social structures of Finnish society changed rapidly, moving away from agrarianism and toward industrialization. Family structures were also shaped by this process of modernization. The number of households including family members from more than two generations decreased, and the amount of so called "nuclear families" increased. Nuclear families consist of only two generations and do not include grandparents. The divorce rate also increased remarkably between the 1960s and the late 1990s, before stabilizing at approximately 50 per cent. As a result of these changes, the roles of grandparents in children's lives were altered.

The role of grandparents in child care has diminished; however, kinship relationships continue to be an important part of many people's everyday lives. The basic line of kinship help in Finnish families' moves from parents to younger generations, which most people take for granted (Haavio-Mannila et al., 2009). Regardless of this fact, grandparents in Finland do not have any official status, grandparenthood is not supported by social policy, and there is no statutory regulation governing the rights and duties of grandparents. Each separate case must be processed with regard to the best interests of the child. The Finnish Child Welfare Act (417/2007) requires the network of people close to the child to be identified as part of the process, stating that "before a child's placement away from home, it is necessary to investigate what opportunities there are for the child to live with the parent with whom the child does not primarily reside, with the relatives or with other persons close to the child, or for these parties otherwise to participate in supporting the child," and adds that this process "may be omitted if it is not required on account of the urgency of the case or for some other justified reason." It also emphasizes that "the child's accommodation or placement location must always be resolved in a manner consistent with the child's interests" (Child Welfare Act 417/2007, Article 32).

Kinship care is an important topic in the field of child welfare and, following political debate, is viewed as a growing trend in the field of foster care and child custody. There are great differences in the views of social workers on kinship foster parenting, meaning that there is wide variation in the practices of awarding custody of a child to relatives in cases where parents are deemed incapable (Heino, 2001). There are no exact statistics about kinship care in Finland, but it is known that roughly less than a fifth of all foster parenting cases and less than a tenth of all custody cases are kinship custodies. Significant differences exist between kinship foster families involving grandparents and those involving other relatives, in terms of age, health, education, profession, family income, and type of housing, as well as in motives for kinship foster parenting (Koisti-Auer, 2008).

As a result of the lack of relevant regulations, grandparents in Finland can only gain custody or become foster parents if the court finds that this is in the best interest of a child. The municipal welfare body responsible for social services is also responsible for taking measures to arrange the care of a child, by agreement between the parents, or by a court decision if this is deemed appropriate in view of the child's interests. These decisions also concern the adoption of children by their grandparents. According to the Adopt Act, the adoption of a child "may be granted if it is deemed to be in the best interests of the child and if it has been established that the child will be well taken care of and brought up." The act states that "a petition for the granting of adoption shall contain proof that the child is in the care of the adopter or that the latter is otherwise in charge of the care and upbringing of the child" (Adopt Act 153/1985, Section 2).

A Social Worker Responds

There are 2,810 HIV positive adults in Finland, out of a population of 5.4 million people (Handbook of Nursing, 2011). Therefore, this case must be addressed hypothetically. Although there are few HIV positive children in Finland, there are child abuse cases on which to base the role of the social workers in our analysis.

In Finland, social work plays a major role in several fields involved in our case. These include social work in local social offices (including child protection and family law affairs), the health care system, and the police department. Each of these would work with Ruth and the grandfather in question. Social workers would undoubtedly have known the girl in this case before the criminal occurrence, because of her being orphaned and suffering a serious illness; they would already be making a significant contribution in the girl's life. The following section outlines the main functions of social work in the life of Ruth, her mother, and Sam both before and after the crime is committed.

First, all pregnant women come under the care of prenatal and child health clinics. If a pregnant woman is diagnosed with HIV or AIDS, she is directed to a special health care service where she would meet a social worker. The administration of medication to prevent the child from being infected with the HI virus would begin immediately. The social worker would be in contact with the woman's home municipality, and the mother and child would become clients of the local child protection agency (so-called "antici-pating child protection"). A plan of support activities needed by the family would be drawn up in collaboration with personnel from social and health care services (housing, living, health), and a social worker would work with the family before the child was born.

The second issue is that, according to Finnish law, the custody of a child must be determined officially when the single parent/mother is dead. A grandparent can apply for custody of the child from a local court. According to the law, the relatives can become the custodians of a child if it is in his or her best interest (Child Welfare Act, 2007, Section 50), with the local social office responsible for the assessment (ibid, Section 81). Currently in Finland, more than 16,000 children are placed at any one time, and less than 10 per cent are with relatives (Känkänen & Laaksonen, 2006; Official Statistics of Finland, 2010). In this case, the situation of the biological father would be determined, if possible, from the point of view of custody. Thereafter, the local court would request official help from the social security office to investigate the circumstances, which is a requirement for making a decision concerning custody. A local social worker would conduct the investigation, and then make an official statement to the local court. In the case in question, it can be assumed that the grandfather was found suitable to have custody of his grandchild. From the psychosocial point of view, it would be important for a vulnerable child to maintain a permanent and safe attachment to her grandfather and possibly with other members of her extended family at the same time (Howe, 2005).

In this case, suitable support would have been provided for the grandfather, according to his needs. It can be assumed that Sam is retired and therefore, in addition to his pension, he would receive financial support from the local social security office to cover costs of the custody (reward for family care), child benefit fixed by law, and support for child-rearing activities from the family counseling system.

Third, Ruth is always a client of the social work department when involved in a criminal investigation. In this case, social workers from the police department, health care system, and local child protection office would have dealt with the matter. When the child initially went to the hospital for examination, she would have met a social worker who would report the offence to the police if the grandfather had not already done so. The social worker or a doctor would contact the forensic psychiatric investigation unit for children and young people which is present in all university hospitals. The units are staffed by child and youth psychiatrists, psychologists, and social workers who specialize in investigating crimes against children and young people, such as physical and sexual abuse. The unit's on-call workers would meet the child immediately, if needed. Otherwise, the investigation of sexual abuse will start later when the police send an official request for investigation.

The law stipulates that there must be a forensic psychiatric investigation of child sexual abuse. It is part of the process of preliminary crime investigation and must be carried out in collaboration with the family, police authorities, and social workers from the police department and the local child protection system. However, the investigation process starts at the request of the police authorities (Criminal Code 1889, Chapters 20 and 21) and is carried out by specially trained doctors, psychologists, and social workers, with the government covering 80 per cent of the cost. The process consists of a network meeting (including police, representatives of child protection, and other relevant quarters); somatic investigations, if needed; one or two forensic psychological interviews; psychological investigations (cognitive/personality); a child psychiatric individual investigation; interviews with parents; interaction assessments, if needed; a statement to the police department; guiding the child through follow-up care; and testifying in court when requested. The forensic child and youth psychiatric unit makes a statement to the police about the probability of a crime having been committed and the plausibility of the story of the child, assesses the level of damage and the need for care, and organizes follow-up care.

The task of social workers within the forensic psychiatric unit is to interview the adult members of the family about what happened and to investigate the living conditions, history, interaction, and social networks of the family. The social worker contacts local social workers in the family's home area to consider the living conditions of the child and the need for child protection activities. The fundamental task of the social worker in the forensic psychiatric unit is to discover whether the child is safe at the grandfather's home, or if she has a pressing need for somewhere else to live. Accordingly, the social worker would carry out her or his duties as part of this process. After the investigation, the social worker would organize adequate follow-up care, stabilize the child's life situation, and arrange follow-up visits required by the child and her custodians.

As the 11-year-old girl is the victim of serious sexual abuse, it is clear that she will need both psychiatric and social follow-up care. The family will need financial and mental support to continue the task of her upbringing while fulfilling her best interests. The mental support mainly involves therapy and counseling, and it is primarily the task of the local child protection authority to control and organize this support. Social workers play a key role in the Finnish child protection system, but the law obliges all professional groups in all fields and at all levels of society to contribute. A major role of local social workers is to be responsible for child protection, which includes case management in the multi-disciplinary and multi-professional system of welfare services.

The provision of care and the protection of children are viewed as essential parts of the Nordic welfare system. Children and young people are regarded as competent social actors with their own rights to influence their daily lives and society (Eydal & Kröger, 2010, p. 12). This means that a child has a right to be heard and her opinion should be taken into account, especially in decisions concerning personal relations with people close to her. The priority in social work is considering the best interests of the child; therefore, social workers have to protect a child while promoting her participation and provision of resources. In this case, therapy may be required to aid recovery from her traumatic experience.

Case study #3

Transitioning from Home to Institutional Care

BY DUANE LUPTAK FROM THE US

Delia is a 42-year-old woman diagnosed with paranoid schizophrenia and takes medication to help control hallucinations and delusions. She is diagnosed with diabetes and needs to take insulin. She is also morbidly obese. She has never been employed, is functionally illiterate, and can only read and write a few words. She has medical assistance and gets additional income from the government.

Delia was admitted to an inpatient psychiatric unit at a local hospital after her daughters took her to the emergency room saying she was "acting crazy" and that she should not be allowed to return to the apartment because "she can't take care of herself." Delia was expressing thoughts of suicide at the time of her admission to the hospital seven days ago, but is no longer expressing those thoughts and seems ready for discharge back to the community. Delia says she needs a social worker to help her find housing because her landlord is evicting her from the apartment. The lease is terminating at the end of the month (15 days) and her landlord has given her notice that he will not renew her lease. It is a one-bedroom apartment with rent subsidized by the government. She needs to vacate the apartment in 15 days or eviction proceedings will commence.

Delia has two unmarried adult daughters who are both homeless and each has two children. The children range in age from one– four years, and it appears that the daughters and their children have been living with Delia on and off for the past several months. The neighbors have complained to the landlord about the children running unsupervised around the apartment building and about visitors coming and going from the building at all hours of the day and night. Her neighbors say they suspect the daughters are involved with illegal drug use and dealing. Delia has maintained that her family is important to her and she intends to help them however she can. She hopes to stay close with her children and grandchildren when she moves into a facility.

Transitioning from Home to Institutional Care: A Social Worker from Japan Responds

BY YOMEI NAKATANI

Prevalence & Incidence

Japan's elder population continues to increase at an unprecedented rate, and is the highest in the world. Traditionally, the elderly have been cared for by their relatives. As part of Japan's caregiving norms, the elderly are most likely to be cared for by family members, either their own direct kin (mostly women) or in-laws (mostly daughters-in-law). Over time, it has become difficult to maintain this practice due to the fact that most caregivers are themselves growing old. Since the caregiving population is aging, it is difficult for them to perform some of the physically exacting tasks involved. Not many Japanese live in institutional homes, because there is an unfavorable notion about their use. Hospital placement is more acceptable (Ng, 2007).

Country Policies

Japanese welfare policy reflects the traditional ideology of family care. Some of the early laws that provided a framework for elder care in Japan were the 1963 Social Welfare Service Law for the Elderly (Rojin Fukushi Ho) and the 1982 Health and Medical Service Law for the Elderly (Rojin Hoken Ho). With respect to care for seniors, Japanese society generally leaned towards family care and support. This cultural orientation influenced policymaking so that the Social Welfare Service Law for the Elderly focused on low income earners without family support (Ihara, n.d).

Social care for the elderly garnered support in the 1990s, encouraging public acceptance of the use of social services. This acceptance eventually culminated in the Long-Term Care Insurance (LTCI). Still the idea of relying or depending on others outside the family for personal and nursing care proves to be a difficult adjustment for some to make (Ng, 2007). *There are two broad categories of benefits available under the LTCI. These are community care benefits, which include services such as bathing, respite care, and home help, and institutional care benefits, with services such as geriatric care and special nursing homes. Not only is the LTCI making care for elders more accessible, it is also making it more affordable for those of middle and high income status* (Ng, 2007). Eligible persons respond to a questionnaire of 85 items, a computer-based assessment (standardized by the national government), and a review from a panel of experts. This determines the level of care they will receive—community or institutional (Lai, 2001). Funds for the LTCI come from premiums paid by the aforementioned groups, and local and national government taxes. The payment of premiums is integrated into the existing social security payment framework (Lai, 2001). For these services, seniors make a 10 per cent co-payment. Adults aged 40 years and over pay 50 per cent of the remaining funds while government pays the other 50 per cent (Ng, 2007; Tsutsui & Muramatsu, 2007).

In 1989, the government developed a plan to promote and enhance care for the elderly by increasing infrastructure and human resources. This plan was dubbed the Ten-Year Strategy to Promote Health Care and Welfare for the Elderly, and was renamed the New Gold Plan in 1994 with a revision of certain targets such as increasing the number of people who offered support to seniors in their homes, and expanding services rendered to seniors in their homes with the inclusion of visits by medical staff (Ihara, n.d; Japan Fact Sheet, n.d).

Care for the elderly received a further boost with the formulation of the LTCI, approved by the Diet (Japan's bicameral legislature) in 1997. Though implemented in 2000, work on the LTCI began with policy deliberations about care for seniors which went on for a number of years (Lai, 2001). Since it is a mandatory insurance policy, all persons (40 years and older) with incomes pay premiums, and older persons (65 years and older) qualify to receive benefits based on their mental and physical disability. People aged 40 to 64 years with age-related disabilities such as Parkinson's or Alzheimer's disease also qualify to receive benefits. The benefits are in the form of services with no cash assistance. The LTCI reflects the transformation in Japan's elder care tradition. It is apparent that the state is assuming what used to be the responsibility of the family (Campbell & Ikegami, 2000).

In anticipation of continued increase in the adult population over 65 years of age and the subsequent need for more services, Japan formulated another Gold Plan in 2000: Gold Plan 21. It is a five-year plan formulated with the intention of increasing infrastructure and generally strengthening policies for elder care (Japan Fact Sheet, n.d; Japan Association of Geriatric Health Services Facilities, n.d).

A Social Worker Responds

Japanese social workers share some universal perspectives and principles developed by the Western social work field, although Japan is culturally an Eastern society. The ecological perspective, or the concept of "person-in-situation," is commonly shared among social workers in Japan. In Delia's case, social workers would try to understand the situation from this standpoint. For example, they might expect at least four professionals to be involved in this type of case: a psychiatric physician from a hospital or clinic, a district nurse from a local health center, a local officer from a district social welfare agency, and the social worker him/herself. The team would consider a variety of formal and informal networks for Delia such as support from a local welfare agency office, her family and relatives, and friends and neighbors.

The family is an important unit social workers need to consider. Japanese social workers typically see a family as a client system rather than focusing on an individual, probably because the Japanese social work field has not experienced a period of engaging deeply in counseling-oriented interventions. In this case, Delia is not only a person who needs help and support—her two daughters are in need as well. Their children too are included in this client system.

In 2003, the Japanese Ministry of Health, Labour and Welfare legally introduced care management services for the mentally ill. The care for Delia would fall under these types of services provisions. Social workers are primarily expected to take on the role of a care manager in the Japanese mental health field. Thus, in Delia's case, a social worker is supposed to lead the case management process.

A social worker would identify at least three different needs in this case. First, Delia needs housing. There may be a possibility of renegotiating with her landlord. However, it is hard to do so since in Japanese society there is still a stigma toward the mentally ill. Second, Delia's daughters and their children need a place to settle. Because Delia's apartment is subsidized by the government, they cannot keep the place when Delia's lease terminates. Third, Delia and her daughters' families need to live close to one another. The daughters and their children are something to live for in Delia's life even though she can support them only in a limited fashion.

After identifying the needs in this case, a social worker would plan to set up a care conference, which might include a psychiatric physician from Delia's hospital, a district nurse from a local health center, and a local officer from a district social welfare agency. These people are key service providers for implementing community services for the mentally ill in Japan. A social worker would share information about the case with these professionals, give them information about the identified needs from a social work assessment, and discuss plans to implement needed interventions and services.

Plans to intervene in this case might be established as follows. For Delia's place to live, seeking some type of institutional care seems appropriate. Since she is not familiar with living in long-term facilities, Delia may be placed in a short-term recovery facility to prepare for the move to a long-term care facility. After leaving the recovery facility, a group-care home is her first choice to stay. If she could obtain a job, Delia would be able to find another apartment for rent and receive a variety of community services such as homemaker services so that she could live with her family.

Additionally, a social worker would try to reach other family members since most of the cases in Japan providing care for the mentally ill still consider it the family's job. Simultaneously, Japanese families generally feel *haji* (great shame) when one of the family members suffers from mental illness. Therefore, families may try to hide a patient from neighbors or avoid contact with a patient. According to Delia's life history, it is less realistic to ask her family to work on some part of her care.

A plan for the second need (placing Delia's daughters' families) is to consider a sheltered facility for the mothers and fatherless children. The daughters would need special assistance or guidance due to their possible drug use history. A social worker could arrange counseling services or peer-support services within the sheltered house or utilize services provided outside the house. If a social worker focuses on the issue of appropriate childrearing options for the daughters 'children, it might be considered in the best interests of the children that their guardianship be provided by other persons or a legal entity such as local government. In the Japanese legal system, removing guardianship from a natural parent is rare.

In addressing the third need (keeping Delia in contact with her daughters), a social worker could engage in a variety of activities to connect Delia with her daughters' families. For example, a social worker would arrange to have Delia visit her daughters' sheltered housing and have them visit Delia's group-care home. Also, planning "getting together with the whole family" activities outside their residences, such as shopping or traveling, might be other possible choices.

The Japanese social work profession requires a bachelor's degree level education, not a master's level, although Japan began a national licensure system in 1987. Therefore, social workers are less independent and less able to be creative in their profession when compared to social workers from other countries. Japanese social workers are more dependent on the policies and regulations of agencies or organizations by which they are employed. Since social work is regulated, Japanese social workers can engage actively in case management.

Transitioning from Home to Institutional Care: A Social Worker from Hungary Responds

BY MARTA B. ERDOS, NIKOLETTA MANDI, JOZSEF MADACSY, JOZSEF CSURKE, & GEORGINA MUCSI

Prevalence and Incidence

The rate of employment is 55.4 per cent; and the average net earnings are presently 140,400 HUF. Currently, 499,200 persons receive disability pension; this rate is decreasing as criteria for eligibility have been changed (National Central Statistical Office, n.d.). The prevalence of psychiatric disorders is around 1.5 per cent; with a total of 145,532 patients registered in out-patient treatment centers in 2008 (persons with addictions are not included). In 2010, the incidence was 18,496 (adults with psychiatric disorders) (National Central Statistical Office, n.d.). By 2010, 7,878 persons lived in traditional residential homes, 65 persons in temporary homes, and 310 persons in family-like homes established for 8–12 persons (National Central Statistical Office, n.d.). Approximately 20 per cent of all psychiatric patients are diagnosed with schizophrenia. Mental disorders are a leading cause for disability retirement (National Central Statistical Office, n.d.).

The urban population is 68 per cent of the total population, and the percentage living below the poverty line is 13.9 per cent (CIA World Factbook, 2011). The poverty line (60 per cent of median income) was 59,599 HUF in 2009; and the breadline was 78,730 HUF/one consumption units in 2010. The percentage of those living under the breadline is 37 per cent. An important measure determining eligibility for the social benefits minimum is the old age pension (28,500 HUF) (Hungarian Central Statistical Office, June 2011).

Country Policies

Until the communist bureaucracy eliminated social work as a profession on ideological grounds soon after the Soviet invasion of Hungary in 1945, the development of social work in Hungary followed certain Western trends and worked out its own solutions to specific problems (Zimmermann, 1997). Communists considered social policy and social work unnecessary. According to Marxist-Leninist ideology, all deviances, including mental disorders, were determined to be the results of exploitation. The system claimed itself to be free from exploitation; consequently, identification and treatment of many mental and social problems were not possible until the late 1970s. This ideology seriously hindered the development of the helping professions, including psychiatry, clinical psychology, and social work.

The legalization of the helping and social professions began some years before the transition to the current social system in 1989. Psychiatric patients needing residential care lived in rural settlements at a great distance from their previous communities. The system strived to colonize citizens' entire life-worlds and employed various means of control. Political psychiatry (misusing diagnosis and treatment for political purposes) was among the central mechanisms, but treatment in a hospital might as well have served as an escape for some political "deviants" (Erdos, 2006).

By the 1970s, mental problems for many people grew, and Hungary experienced high rates of suicide and alcoholism (Elekes & Skog, 1993). The system, previously a barrier for the development of psychiatric care, organized its first models according to party hierarchy. These models did not address the mental health issues faced by a number of Hungarians.

One relative advantage of the state socialist era was that Hungary's health care system worked independently of financial interests. The 1980s brought a boom in psychotherapeutic methods with the Hungarian professionals following Western trends; however, they were also developing their own approaches and specializations. Social work as a profession has only recently been included in the areas of medical care. Deinstitutionalization occurred concurrently with the social transition. Large and alienating institutions as central elements of psychiatric care were exchanged for community care. Presently, in spite of the possible benefits, these new forms are still under-represented in the system, due to serious financing problems.

Today, psychiatry is largely dominated by biomedical approaches. For the social professionals working in the field, hierarchic relations and lack of public recognition are a major challenge, but there are some promising examples of inter-professional collaboration. However, clinical social worker competencies and tasks have not yet been clearly defined.

The global financial crisis hit Hungary hard: disability pensions were considerably reduced, with a number of people being re-qualified as "healthy enough" and no longer entitled to disability pensions. Many people with psychiatric problems and a history of decades of unemployed status were urged to find employment. A large number of people with psychiatric problems have incomes far below the Hungarian breadline. Recent data are not available, but the number of people living below this level is on the rise. The rate of (registered) unemployment is currently around 11 per cent in the country and clients do not have a chance in the open labor market. Protected workplaces are hard to find and rehabilitation work is an opportunity mostly for those living in a residential home.

Country policies are shaped by Act III (1993) and Ministerial Decree no. 1 (2000) (Ministry of Social and Family Affairs), which determines the possible (but not always accessible) forms of care provided for patients with psychiatric disorders. The basic level of care includes providing daily meals, family help, home care (less than 4 hours/day in the client's own home), community care, and daytime care. Second level specialized (residential) care forms include:

- In-patient rehabilitation facility where training, work activities and other forms of therapy are organized and patients should be prepared for their return to the community;
- Transitory homes for the patients who do not need permanent medical care or a residential home but, momentarily, the family cannot provide the necessary care for them. The capacity is only 100 in Hungary and the service is not available in the Southern-Transdanubian Region;
- Residential homes for psychiatric patients: the patient needs more than 4 hours/day permanent support in accomplishing daily tasks. Referral is based on the regional psychiatrist's expert opinion;
- Family-like homes: availability is restricted due to financial problems.

A specific feature of the Hungarian system is that both legal regulations and professional approaches (organizational models and expertise) would facilitate a high-level of care for patients, but severe financial limitations are often imposed on the system. What is legally or theoretically outlined is not actually available; and the result is that some patients with psychiatric disorders will live part of their lives in the institutions for homeless persons, the cheapest form of social care in Hungary. Very often, the availability of an institution depends on the social worker's informal professional connections; that is, when the social worker encounters a patient, it is not the protocol but the social worker's social capital that is decisive in the helping process. Regional inequality of access to the services is also present.

A Social Worker Responds

In Hungary, rent is not subsidized by the government. Delia could not live on her own unless she owned the apartment. As disability pensions and other benefits have been reduced recently, she could easily become indebted and would now face the danger of homelessness. It is unlikely that this is Delia's first contact with a social worker if she never worked before and lived on disability pension, social benefits, and allowances.

The hospital social worker would first explore her network of social relationships (i.e., other relatives, acquaintances, and the professionals who have helped her so far). He/she would immediately contact the local Psychiatric Rehabilitation Ward and ask for Delia's admission. He/she would have to ask this as a personal favor, and promise that Delia's case will be solved in a few months. Also, he/she would notify the Child Welfare Service to assess if Delia's grandchildren are abused. This service would determine if any form of professional assistance is sufficient and available for Delia's daughters to enable them to properly care for their children.

Although there is no immediate danger of self-harm, Delia's somatic problems may indicate that she requires further medical supervision and more control of her psychotropic medication for possible side effects (diabetes and obesity are often a sign of such problems). Second, due to long waiting lists in residential care and the client's pressing situation, a few months in a rehabilitation ward may save Delia from homelessness. Although Delia has never worked, the social worker would attempt to find Delia some rehabilitation employment. At the rehabilitation ward, the staff would assess her abilities and motivation, as well as help her to become accustomed to structuring her day.

Disability pensions and other social benefits are low in Hungary; if she is relying solely on these, Delia would not be able to live on her own. If her daughters are in fact involved in illegal drug use, they need help and cannot support their mother effectively. For lack of workplaces in the labor market and the client's serious health problems, Delia would have go into residential care after leaving the rehabilitation ward. The length of rehabilitation treatment is determined more by the length of the waiting list at the residential home than Delia's health status. Since the homes are in small villages and commuting is expensive and time-consuming, contact with her family would probably lessen, but she would be safe.

Another alternative is community care (daytime center and frequent contacts with the social worker); however, Delia's safety could be at risk here. Housing is the most difficult problem, but Delia could stay close to her children and grandchildren. The social worker should inform Delia about the consequences of both alternatives and, by understanding her potential, prospects, and social network, should help her decide and prepare for the changes in her life. Delia's own wishes should be respected as much as is possible under the given circumstances. For Delia and her Hungarian social worker, the dilemma of the case is between safety and connectedness.

Exercises

In Class

The following exercises are for in-class discussion.

- Describe what you would do if you were the social worker for any one of these cases. Compare how that response would be different from/similar to the responses provided. Why would your response be different from/similar to the responses provided?
- Consider the role of social service agencies in working with the elderly. What are the resources available in your area?
- How do men and women experience aging? What are the main social welfare issues that they face?
- Locate information from your city/county/state/country about the elderly. What types of data are available? What issues are facing the elderly? How can social work interventions assist with these issues?

Outside of Class

For each of the exercises below, select a country different from your home country and the countries discussed in this chapter. Present your findings to your peers in class.

- Search for sources in another country that provide information about aging and the issues facing the elderly. Summarize what the resources are and where they are located.
- Consider the laws in another country that deal with elder abuse and neglect. Compare the laws to those in your home country. Who do the laws protect? Why?
- Conduct a thorough literature search about the impact of aging and caregiving in one or two countries. Draft a summary about the information you find on this topic.
- Develop a list of agencies in your country that could support the elderly. What are the mission statements of these agencies? How are

the statements linked to actual practice for social workers? Is there a different set of agencies for dealing with the very old (people 85 years and older)?

- Interview one or two of your social work peers about their knowledge of social work practice and working with the elderly. Ask them about the incidence of and community attitudes toward services for aging populations.

References

Act III of 1993 on Social Governance and Social Benefits (Finland)

Administration on Aging (2011). Retrieved from http://www.aoa.gov/AoARoot/ AoA_Programs/HCLTC/Caregiver/index.aspx Adopt Act 153/1985. Finland

Adopt Act 153/1985. Finland.

Antikainen, J. (2005). "Seksuaalisesti hyväksikäytettyjen lasten hoito ja nuorten hyväksikäyttäjien auttaminen. Kirjallisuuskatsaus." [Helping and treatment of sexually abused children and sexually abusive young people] Stakes työpapereita 13. Helsinki.

Antonucci, T. C., Okorodudu, C., & Akiyama, H. (2002). "Well–being among older adults on different continents." *Journal of Social Issues*, 58, 617–26.

Baker, L. A., Silverstein, M., Putney, N.M. (2008). "Grandparents raising grandchildren in the US: changing family forms, stagnant social policies." *Journal of Social Policy*, 7, 53–69.

Campbell, J., & Ikegami, N. (2000). Long-term care insurance comes to Japan. *Health Affairs, 19(3)*, 26–39.

Child Welfare Act (2007). The Child Welfare Act of Finland 417/2007.

Conference on psychosocial counseling. Group discussion. SANSZ-TAMOP –5.5.1/A-10/1-2010-0011, Pecs.

Criminal Code 1889. The Criminal Code of Finland 39/1889. Chapter 20: Sex offences (563/1998). Chapter 21: Homicide and bodily injury (578/1995).

Cuddy, A. C., Norton, M. I., & Fiske, S. T. (2005). "This old stereotype: The pervasiveness and persistence of the elderly stereotype." *Journal of Social Issues*, 61, 267–85.

Davies, E., & Higginson, I. J. (Eds.) (2004). "Better palliative care for older people." World Health Organization, Regional Office for Europe. Retrieved from http://www.euro.who.int/__data/assets/pdf_file/0009/98235/E82933.pdf

Elekes, Zs. & Skog, O.J. (1993). "Alcohol and the 1950–90 Hungarian Suicide trend – Is There a Casual Connection?" *Acta Sociologica*, 36, 33–46.

Erdos, M. B. (2006). A *nyelvben elo kapcsolat* [The Language Bond]. Budapest: Typotex.

Eydal, G. B. & Kröger, T. (2010). "Nordic Family Policies: Constructing Contexts for Social Work with Families." In H. Forsberg & T. Kröger (Eds.) *Social work and child welfare politics*. Through Nordic Lenses. Bristol: Policy Press, pp. 11–27.

Feldman, S. & Damron-Rodriguez, J. (2007). "The art of adapting to health challenges with age: Introduction." In S. Carmel, C. A. Morse, & F. M. Torres-Gil (Eds.). *Lessons on aging from three nations, volume i: The art of aging well.* Amityville, NY: Baywood Publishing Company Inc.

Goodman, C. C., Potts, M. K., Pasztor, E. M. (2007) "Caregiving grandmothers with vs. without child welfare system involvement: effects of expressed need, formal services, and informal social support on caregiver burden." *Child and Youth Services Review*, 29, 428–41.

Haavio-Mannila, E., Majamaa, K., Tanskanen, A., Hämäläinen, H., Karisto A., Rotkirch, A., & Roos, J. P. (2009). "Sukupolvien ketju. Suuret ikäluokat ja sukupolvien välinen vuorovaikutus Suomessa." [A Chain of Generations. Baby Boomers and Cross-Generational Interaction in Finland] Sosiaali- ja terveysturvan tutkimuksia 107. Helsinki: Kela.

Handbook of Nursing (2011). "HIV-hoitotyön käsikirja. 3 uudistettu painos." Helsinki: Helsinki University Hospital.

Heino, Tarja (2001). "Sijoitukset sukulaisperheisiin lastensuojelussa." [Placements into Kinship Families in Child Welfare] Aiheita 19/2001. Helsinki: Stakes.

Howe, D. (2005). *Child Abuse and Neglect: Attachment, Development and Intervention.* London: Palgrave/Macmillan.

Hungarian Central Statistical Office (2011). Retrieved from http://www.ksh.hu/?lang=en

Japan Association of Geriatric Health Services Facilities (n.d.). Retrieved from http://www.roken.or.jp/english.htm

Japan Fact Sheet (n.d.). Welfare for older people. Retrieved from http://web-japan.org/factsheet/en/pdf/e43_welfare.pdf

Känkänen, P., & Laaksonen, S. (2006). "Selvitys sijaishuollon ja jälkihuollon nykytilasta ja kehittämistarpeista." Lastensuojelun kehittämisohjelma.

Koisti-Auer, A.-L. (2008). "Sukulaisvanhemmuuden profiili." [Profile of Kinship Care] Tutkimuksia 1/2008. Jyväskylä: Pesäpuu ry.

Lai, O.K. (2001). Long-term care policy reform in Japan. *Journal of Aging & Social Policy, 13(2/3)*, 5–20.

Lamanna, M. A., & Riedmann, A. (2006). *Marriages & Families: Making Choices and Facing Change.* Belmont, CA: Thomson/Wadsworth.

Laaksonen, T., Sariola, H., Johansson, A., Jern, P., Varjonen, M., von der Pahlen, B., Sandnabba, N. K., & Santtila, P. (2011). "Changes in the prevalence of child sexual abuse, its risk factors, and their associations as a function of age cohort in a Finnish population sample." *Child Abuse & Neglect*, 35 (7), 480–90.

Lent, J. P. (2005). "Grandparents and other relatives raising children: a primer for the KIDS COUNT network." Retrieved from www.kidscount.org/kcnetwork/resources/documents/Grandparentsbackgroundpaperfinal.doc

Long-Term Care Insurance Benefit for the Elderly in Korea. Retrieved from http://www.nhic.or.kr/english/healthins/healthins03.htm

Long-term Care Portal South Korea. Retrieved from http://www.longtermcare. or.kr/portal/longtermcare/main.jsp

Ministerial Decree no. 1 (2000) on Professional Tasks of Social Institutions Providing Personal Care, Article 1.7, Ministry of Social and Family Affairs.

Ministry of Health and Welfare Korea (2009). Retrieved from http://english. mw.go.kr/font_eng/index.jsp

National Alliance for Caregiving (2009). Retrieved from http://www.caregiving.org

National Family Caregiver Support Program (2000). Retrived from http://www. agingcarefl.org/caregiver/NationalSupport

National Health Insurance Program South Korea. Retrieved from http://www. nhic.or.kr/english/main.html

Ng, G.T. (2007). Learning from Japanese experience in aged care policy. *Asian Social Work and Policy Review, 1*, 36–51.

Sariola, H. & Uutela, A. (1994). The prevalence and context of child sexual abuse in Finland. *Child Abuse and Neglect 18 (10)*, 827–835.

Sariola, H. &Uutela, A. (1996). The prevalence and context of incest abuse in Finland. *Child Abuse and Neglect 20(9)*, 843–850.

Tsutsui, T., & Muramatsu, N. (2007). Japan's universal long-term care system reform of 2005: Containing costs and realizing a vision. *Journal of the American Geriatrics Society, 55(9)*, 1458–1463.

UN study of violence against children (2006). Retrieved from http://www. unicef.org/violencestudy/reports/SG_violencestudy_en.pdf

US Census (2007). American Community Survey. Retrieved from http://www. census.gov/acs/www/

Waterston, T. & Mok, J. (2008). "Violence against children: the UN report. Archives of Disease in Childhood", 93 (1), 85–8.

Zimmermann, S. (1997). *Prachtige Armut. Fursorge, Kinderschutz und Sozialreform in Budapest. Das "sozialpolitische Laboratorium" der Doppelmonarchie im Vergleich zu Wien 1873–1914* [Splendid Poverty. Poor Relief, Child Provision, and Social Reform in Budapest. The "Social Laboratory" of the Habsburg Monarchy Compared to Vienna 1873–1914]. Historische Forschungen. Im Auftrag der Historischen Kommission der Akademie der Wissenschaften und der Literatur, vol. 21. Sigmaringen: Thorbecke Verlag.

7 Changes in Caregivers

By Joanna E. Bettmann

Several factors have precipitated the need for changes in caregiving for children. These include epidemics, such as HIV and AIDS, ethnic and regional conflicts and natural disasters such as earthquakes. The population of children in the world orphaned by AIDS alone is staggering. Data estimates indicate that, as of 2009, over 16 million children had lost either one or both parents as a result of HIV/AIDS (UNICEF, 2011). Increasing poverty and other socio-economic conditions, as well as congenital diseases and disabilities, also account for the placement of children in institutional care in countries across the world (UNICEF CEECIS, n.d).

Case study #1

Orphans and Orphan Care

BY TSHEPO MOGAPI FROM BOTSWANA

Mary, a 70-year-old grandmother, is raising her grandchild Timothy who is nine years old and HIV positive. Mary is also raising three other school-aged grandchildren and living with two of her adult children who are unemployed. She herself is unemployed and all the family members depend on the food assistance the government provides to the family for the grandchildren. The family also faces a housing problem. They only have two small huts, constructed from cow dung and thatched with grass, which are too small for this family of seven. Mary finds it difficult to take Timothy for monthly medical checkups and to get his medication from the clinic, as the clinic is far from where they live.

Mary possesses very little knowledge about HIV and AIDS. She says she only knows that when an individual has the virus, he or she will eventually die. She is not aware of the risks of transmission. She also notes that she does not remember any essential information that was provided during the HIV education lessons she attended because she was grieving at that time for the recent loss of her adult child, Timothy's mother. At times, she receives transport from the government home-based care program to go to the clinic to collect the medication, and at times she also receives assistance in the form of money and food from her son who works in a major city. The family has not disclosed Timothy's HIV status to anyone because they believe it is their family's secret. They tell their neighbors that Timothy is suffering from chest problems whenever he is not well.

Mary is pleased to be raising Timothy since she feels it is her responsibility to care for him. She enjoys Timothy's company, and says that he is a well-behaved child. The family's socio-economic circumstances and its inability to reveal the truth of Timothy's illness to the community is a big setback. It means that they are not receiving all the support that would be possible if others were aware of their plight. The clinic at which Timothy receives care encourages them to consult with the clinic's social worker.

Orphans and Orphan Care: A Social Worker from Bulgaria Responds

BY DIMITRINKA BUMBOVSKA & RITTA ROSANITA SIMONIA

Prevalence and Incidence

The Republic of Bulgaria has a population of more than seven million; about 1,360,000 of them are children. Currently, about 1,000 children live in residential care. In 11,000 families, children without parents live with their relatives. In 2010, 950 orphaned children were adopted, 300 of them abroad.

Country Policies

Child protection in Bulgaria is assured by the state and implemented by governmental agencies with the involvement of the local authorities/munic-ipalities, non-governmental and private organizations, individuals, local communities, and the general public. The responsibilities of all the parties involved in child protection are regulated by the Bulgarian Child Protection

Act (2000), Family Code (2009), Social Support Act (1998), and other legislation. According to these regulations, numerous governmental agencies and the mayors are responsible for child protection in Bulgaria. Under the regulations of the United Coordination Mechanism (section 6a, paragraph 3 of the Child Protection Act, April 2010), they are obligated to cooperate in order to provide prevention, protection, and monitoring for children.

The Bulgarian Child Protection Department (CPD) is a key institution for childcare and protection. It is a department in the structure of governmental bodies, located in the main municipalities. The Adoption Council is a unit at this department. Its function includes keeping records of all children in the region to be adopted and of all parents who are candidates for adoption. It mediates between families and children to be adopted, and is also involved in the legal adoption process. Child Protection Departments (CPDs) evaluate candidates and register them. The CPDs are responsible not only for the protection of the children within the family (prevention, reintegration), but also for protection in such situations as placement with relatives, foster families, in residential care, and adoption.

Twenty years ago, lots of children with disabilities were raised in residential care, not in families. For the past ten years, the basic belief of Bulgarian childcare policy has been that the best interest of the child is to be raised in the family; residential care is a last resort. Due to this shift, the number of children in residential care decreased, but the number of foster families is rising.

Social workers in Bulgaria qualify to practice after completing a four-year Bachelor's degree program at a university. The status of the profession is not high as salaries are rather low; but in recent years, public awareness of the profession has grown. There is no system for certification or licensing social workers in Bulgaria. As soon as they get their university degree, social workers are considered qualified to practice social work.

A Social Worker Responds

If they seek assistance, Mary and Timothy could go to the CPD in their neighborhood or to an NGO that provides social services for families and children. If the family does not seek help or refuses it, medical staff at the hospital will inform the local CPD. According to the Child Protection Act, Timothy is considered a child at risk and thus has the right to be protected and provided with proper care and services. A meeting with the family might be organized at the medical office, where a social worker from the CPD would be present. During the meeting, the social worker would try to build a relationship of trust with the clients and convince them to visit the

CPD office where they could receive counseling, and a variety of benefits and social services, or be directed to other providers of adequate social services.

The social worker will not try to convince the grandmother to share her pain with the neighbors because he/she is aware of the potential shame, fear, and social isolation associated with an HIV diagnosis. Nevertheless, the social worker will try to convince the grandmother to share her pain with the social worker or a psychologist, so as to be understood and supported. Her confidentiality will be assured and her privacy protected.

Timothy is HIV positive and his medical problems indicate the possibility of AIDS. If he is registered for a "disability level" with the government, the family could receive disability benefits and social services. The "disability level" is the percentage of working capability that is lost (above 50, 70, or 90), and the reduced social adaptability of a person. The percentage is determined under Health Ministry regulations and is given by an authorized medical commission on the basis of required medical tests. The social worker might also educate Mary about government programs that could provide day care for Timothy at his home. If Mary prefers to take care of her grandson by herself, she could receive government benefits for doing so.

The social worker should conduct several family home visits that will help him/her to evaluate the problems of the child and his family, decide how to address them, and to meet Timothy's needs for housing, personal space, food, water, heat, electricity, clothes, health care, education, emotional and psychological support, family care, and transportation.

Then the social worker will develop an action plan which should meet all the needs of the child. The social worker will arrange a multi-professional team, consisting of representatives of various government institutions. They will be practitioners of other helping professions (medical staff, teachers, psychologists, lawyers, staff from NGOs, and others). The CPD will present the case to the multi-professional team. Then the action plan developed will be discussed within the team. The main concern of the social worker will be to reach an agreement with the client, his family, and all participants involved in the action plan.

The municipal company provides transport on request to ill people. Thus, the company can provide scheduled transportation to the hospital according to the dates of the medical visits. The municipality could provide municipal housing for the family and thus better living conditions (more rooms, sanitary facilities, cold and hot water, electricity, etc.).

Until financial stabilization of the family occurs, the CPD or other organizations can provide financial support to the family to pay the municipal housing rent. The CPD could also provide financial benefits to cover transportation costs to the hospital. According to state regulations, a family with a child at risk could receive such benefits four times per year which, in total, is an amount of 325 leva (about US $230).

The state pays for the antiretroviral therapy, but the medications must be taken within a precise schedule for optimal results. The hospital will prepare the documents to be presented to the Regional Medical Commission to obtain a level of disability certificate for Timothy. The commission's decision on level of disability opens the possibility for more effective medical treatment of the child and ensures finance for it.

The Local Inspectorate of Education will issue a recommendation for a suitable school for Timothy. Additionally, Timothy could visit a day care center for children with disabilities or special needs. In most cases, the action plan is for six months up to one year. A regular meeting (every three months) of the multi-professional team should be held in order to monitor the implementation of the plan. In the meantime, the CPD will execute a child protection measure for Timothy's "placement with relatives" or "adoption." These measures are not urgent, but to be accomplished they need observation, evaluation, psychological work, and follow up of the progress.

If she decides to take care of Timothy under the "placement at relatives" measure each month, Mary will receive several government-provided benefits: 70 levas (US $50) for raising a child; 168 levas (US $120) for raising a child with disabilities (which is (a) 75 per cent of the minimum monthly wage in Bulgaria); and benefit for raising a foster child—227.50 levas (US $162) in the case of a nine-year-old.

The CPD will monitor the relationship between Mary and her grandson and will consider if she would like to adopt him. According to the Family Code in Bulgaria, Timothy can be adopted by his grandmother. Mary will be advised to put a legal adoption application to the City Court through the Regional Social Support Directorate. In case of adoption, Timothy and Mary will continue to receive the financial, psychological, pedagogical, and legal assistance provided by the CPD.

This particular case requires various institutions to coordinate it. Success depends on the efforts of many professionals, but mainly the social worker from CPD as he/she is the main coordinator in this chain of governmental, municipal, and non-governmental organizations.

Orphans and Orphan Care: A Social Worker from New Zealand Responds

BY MARGARET MCKENZIE

Prevalence and Incidence of the Issue

In New Zealand, the prevalence of HIV/AIDS infection in the general population is very low by international standards. The rate for newly diagnosed cases is stabilizing annually (New Zealand Ministry of Health, 2010). HIV and AIDS awareness, education, and service provision is based on a health promotion and prevention approach, often targeting specific communities.

The prevalence of orphans in Aotearoa New Zealand is low. Aotearoa New Zealand child welfare policy is to ensure whenever possible that children in this situation are living within kinship settings. Foster care is only considered as an option after *whanau* (extended family) and kinship avenues have been exhausted. In some instances, group homes are provided for specialist intervention programs, but always with a Permanency Plan for care beyond the setting.

Aotearoa New Zealand operates a child welfare model based on the support and strengthening of family attachment and engagement. Care for orphaned or unsupported children is provided first and foremost within kinship care frameworks. Welfare benefits and entitlements, the orphans benefit, and unsupported child benefit are targeted at this group.

Country Policies

There are approximately 6,000 social workers nationwide in New Zealand. The largest employer of social workers is the government's child welfare agency: Child, Youth and Family. Additionally social workers can be found in health, justice, and education sectors, and in community-based organizations. A strong voluntary professional membership association, Aotearoa New Zealand Association of Social Workers, has existed since the early 1960s. Their memberships of around 3,000 practitioners are registered under The Social Workers Registration Act of 2003 which introduced voluntary registration. Currently, a discussion paper canvassing mandatory registration is under consideration in New Zealand and the prevailing view is that mandatory registration will be implemented. University education in social work began in the mid-1960s and is now widely available. The basic registerable qualification, Bachelor of Social Work, is a three- or four-year program, depending on the institution.

A Social Worker Responds

In formulating a response from an Aotearoa New Zealand perspective, I chose to focus on aspects of this case where we would act in a way particular to Aotearoa New Zealand, where the issue would fall within child welfare concerns with overlapping issues of risk, protection, health, and well-being.

In Aotearoa New Zealand social work, there is little focus on orphan care. While adoption remains an area within the field of child welfare, the nature of this work has changed significantly in recent decades. In the mid-1970s in New Zealand, the introduction of a government benefit, the Domestic Purposes Benefit for single mothers, enabled a shift towards more women keeping children, and reflected an attitudinal change in society towards acceptance of the practice where stranger care was no longer considered a good option for children.

Consequently fewer and fewer children are available for adoption. Then in 1979, The Children, Young Persons and Their Families Act was passed. This legislation provided a paradigmatic shift in thinking about child welfare provisions. It reinforced the principles of family care and family decision making through strengthening and maintaining kinship or *whanau* involvement for children in need of care and protection. It was underpinned by an acceptance of Maori principles of valuing and foregrounding ongoing kinship connection and kin involvement for childcare, protection and well-being decisions, planning and provision. It is widely accepted as a way forward in addressing the cycle of ongoing negative outcomes for Maori children who were predominantly placed in stranger and European care up until this point.

Central to the approach of child and family social workers in Aotearoa New Zealand is the intention to work from a "doing with," rather than a "doing to" perspective. "Doing with" involves bringing together cooperative partnerships between families, communities, and government, a process of working with and not imposing on. The first concern in this situation would be to engage the family so that the social worker could collaboratively work alongside family members to maximize both their family capital and community networks. Such relational practice (Morris & Burford, 2007) is core to achieving an understanding of the family's capacities and experiences to enable them to access the maximum support available. This can occur through family meetings where all members are invited to be present and participate, including the children.

The social worker would first recognize the strengths and resources that exist within this family group. It appears there is a family desire to keep the situation secret; coupled with a lack of detailed knowledge about Timothy's HIV positive condition that hampers the ability of the family to receive assistance. Thus a careful acknowledgment of this situation is important in building rapport. The question worth asking is "How has this happened?"

Listening to the stories of loss and dislocation that already exist in the family must come first. By attending to the unique aspects of their story, the social worker hopes the family will give up their initial resistance and begin to open up. This active listening can help the worker identify and build upon resources in the family. For example, the supports and resources that already exist include the son who sends money and the clinic (though used only occasionally). Other supports and resources that could be accessed include available adults in the kin network, clinic staff, the social worker, government home care program funding, and community representatives.

Families and communities hold the solutions to their issues. Families do this best when supported by extended family (*whanau*) and by their community. This support helps to reduce and avoid the conflict so characteristic of the traditional adversarial child welfare system. This conceptual framework stresses a full understanding of the capacities and experiences that the family brings, but also notes that the resources available within the welfare system of the region are crucial. The social worker cannot abrogate responsibility but must believe in family participation and family rights at a policy and services level.

Case study #2

Attachment Issues among Children with Multiple Caregivers

BY LAUREN STIVERS & ANDREA RIES FROM THE US

Adam's mother was a single parent who suffered from a substance abuse problem. She used alcohol heavily on a daily basis and frequently was too drunk to take care of her child. When Adam was two, she left him with his grandmother permanently. At the age of three, the grandmother relinquished him to the government's social service department. She said that she couldn't take care of him anymore because he was too much trouble.

She reported that he had tortured small animals, displayed his genitalia frequently to children in their neighborhood, and was defiant and lacked empathy for others.

At this point, the government's social service department contacted Adam's biological mother, who said she missed him and wanted to be with him again. She entered a residential alcohol treatment program where Adam was allowed to live with her at the facility. The staff at the facility reported that Adam had some inappropriate sexual behaviors (displaying himself to others), but overall was a manageable child. The mother, on the other hand, reported being overwhelmed by Adam's care and felt that his behaviors were uncontrollable. Adam's mother left treatment, leaving Adam at the facility.

Adam was placed with a temporary foster home until a family willing to adopt him was located. Although the treatment facility had not reported violence towards animals or other children, the government social worker felt the safest option was to place Adam in a home with no pets and only older siblings. Adam remained in the temporary foster home for four months. The family reported some defiant behaviors, but stated that overall Adam was a pleasure to have around. Another family agreed to adopt Adam and so he moved into another home. Adam lived with this potential adoptive family for eight months. The adoptive mother discovered that Adam had been hiding a knife under his bed. When she confronted him, he physically attacked her. She requested that he be removed immediately from her home.

Adam was now five years old. He was placed back with his first foster family while another potential adoptive family was located. Again, the temporary foster family reported that they enjoyed their time caring for Adam and, although his defiance was at times a challenge, he was a wonderful child. It was made clear to Adam that this family would not be able to adopt him. After a month, Adam was placed with a new potential adoptive family.

Adam was well behaved in his new adoptive home for a month. He then began to have escalating behavior problems and to show verbal and physical aggression and he ran away multiple times. Although the family received family therapy and other help from a social worker, Adam's behavior escalated to the point where the family asked the government's social service department to remove him from the home. Adam was devastated and cried for weeks over this loss. At this point, Adam was about to turn six. He was placed again with the temporary foster family, who expressed an interest in adopting him. Again Adam escalated his behaviors until they were dangerous and unmanageable for the family, and he had to be moved again to another home. He was heartbroken. Finally, his teacher at school became licensed as a foster parent and expressed an interest in adopting Adam. They had bonded at school and she was well aware of his challenges, having heard from his families about the challenges in his homes. She had some training in working with attachment-disordered children, but asked for a social worker's help in assisting Adam to adjusting to his new home with her.

Attachment Issues among Children with Multiple Caregivers: A Social Worker from Ireland Responds

BY MANDI MACDONALD

Prevalence and Incidence

Adam's story is typical of the children currently being adopted in Northern Ireland and across the United Kingdom of Great Britain and Northern Ireland (UK), where the majority of adoptions are of children in care, termed "Looked After Children" (LAC). In 2010, 50 children were adopted from care in Northern Ireland, representing 2 per cent of the "Looked After Children" population (Department of Health, Social Services and Public Safety (DHSSPS), 2011). Of the children who remain in care, the majority of those aged 12 and under are placed with non-kin foster caregivers (64 per cent in 2009), that is with adults who are assessed, approved, and supported by social services to care for a child in their own home, or in foster placements provided by extended family or friends (32 per cent in 2009), while those aged 12 and over are more likely to be looked after in residential children's homes (9 per cent in 2009) (DHSSPS, 2010).

A strong legislative and policy emphasis on keeping children with their birth families means that most adopted children have lived with their birth parents, often with social work support, prior to entering the care system. Many have experience of either trauma or adversity. In a sample of children adopted between 2000 and 2004 in Northern Ireland, 70 per cent were under one year of age when they entered care, while the remainder lived with their birth family up to the age of four before becoming "Looked After" (McSherry et al., 2008). Children are admitted to foster care when they have suffered, or are likely to suffer, significant harm which impairs their health and/or development (Children (NI) Order 1995). Common factors precipitating young children's admission to care include neglect, abuse, domestic violence, parental mental ill-health, and alcohol abuse (McSherry et al., 2008).

Shortages of registered foster families and the crisis nature of some children's family circumstances lead to many foster placements being made as an emergency, necessitating a move when more suitable caregivers are found. Many children also experience unplanned placement disruption, often because caregivers lack the skills and training needed to respond to their complex needs. A survey of children in care in Northern Ireland in 2008–09 showed that almost one quarter (23 per cent) had changed placement at least once in that year, and 3 per cent of those had changed placement three times or more (DHSSPS, 2010).

Once in foster care, extensive efforts are made by social services staff to reunite the child with his/her birth parents before a care plan of adoption can be agreed upon. Therefore, children are rarely adopted in infancy. From entry into foster care, the average length of time for a child to be adopted in 2010 was three years and five months; the average age at adoption was four years and eight months (DHSSPS, 2011).

Attachment difficulties are likely to emerge for many older children adopted from care who have experienced distorted or disrupted relationships with multiple caregivers (Rushton, Monck, Upright & Davidson, 2006). They are also likely to be suffering developmental complications caused by drug/alcohol misuse by their mothers during pregnancy (Northern Ireland Assembly (NIA), 2010), and to have experienced multiple adversity prior to adoption (Rushton et al., 2006). The effects can be enduring, with continuing developmental, behavioral, and social difficulties in evidence up to six years post-adoption (Rushton & Dance, 2004).

Country Policies

Social work in Northern Ireland and throughout the UK is a core element of the welfare state, with the duties and powers of social services departments proscribed by legislation. From its early origins in charitable organizations, social work has become increasingly professionalized. All social workers in the UK must hold a Bachelor's degree in social work and maintain registration with the Northern Ireland Social Care Council (NISCC), which oversees social work education and the conduct of the social care workforce. Social workers practice in health and social care settings operated by government social services departments (statutory), registered charities (voluntary), and private companies, as well as in probation, criminal justice, and education welfare services. Adherence to a common code of ethics, produced by the NISCC, helps ensure consistency of practice.

The central principle which influences Northern Ireland's policies and legislation in relation to social work with children is that every child has a right to belong to a family (NIA, 2010). This principle is based on attachment theory, and enshrined in the United Nations Convention on the Rights of the Child (1989) which was ratified by the UK in 1991. Thus, the thrust of government policy is on enabling children to be cared for by their birth families. The Children (NI) Order 1995 places a duty on social services departments to provide services to prevent children coming into care and to facilitate re-unification with their parents when they do. When children cannot live with their birth families, adoption is viewed as the best alternative for securing stable, permanent family life. This hierarchy of birth family first, adoption second, and other forms of out of home care as a third option, is made explicit in a regional policy on permanency planning for "Looked After Children."

All adoption in Northern Ireland is fully state regulated, and all Health and Social Services Trusts have a statutory duty to provide adoption services. Prospective adopters must be assessed and a registered adoption agency must approve their suitability to adopt and their match with a particular child. When an Adoption Order is made by the Court under the Adoption (NI) Order 1987, the Order affects a complete and irrevocable transfer of legal parentage from the birth parents to the adoptive parents.

Historically, many birth mothers, particularly unmarried mothers, felt constrained by social pressures to relinquish their child for adoption. However, changed social conditions, leading to general acceptance of parenting outside of marriage, mean that very few parents now choose to have their child adopted (O'Halloran, 2001). Indeed, those who do so are likely to experience stigma and guilt (Triseliotis, Feast & Kyle, 2005). Therefore, the majority of adoption proceedings in Northern Ireland are brought to the Court by social services and contested by birth parents. Freeing Orders made under Article 18 of the Adoption (NI) Order, allow for the dispensing of parental consent, and have become the dominant means of securing adoption for children in care in Northern Ireland (Kelly & McSherry, 2003) Because of the far-reaching and permanent effect of a Freeing Order, adoption usually requires an intensive, and often lengthy, process of multi-disciplinary assessment, consultation, and deliberation by the Court.

In Northern Ireland, adoption has come to be seen as a therapeutic intervention for children who have been traumatized by early childhood experiences. But many adopters do not have the skills and specialist knowledge required to provide effective therapeutic parenting (Simmonds, 2008). As the needs and difficulties of children adopted from care are increasingly recognized in policy, practice, and research, there has been a growing emphasis on the need to provide specialist support services for adoptive families. Article 3 of the Adoption (NI) Order places a duty on social services departments to establish and maintain services to meet the needs of adopted children, adopters, and birth parents. New adoptive parents and those fostering with a view to adoption, are entitled to time off from their employment equivalent to maternity leave, and to means-tested adoption allowances payable by government agencies for children who meet certain criteria of need.

A Social Worker Responds

The social worker's role in Adam's case aims to support and consult with the child, to provide support and counseling to his prospective adoptive parent, and to administer the relevant governmental procedures. The social worker would have a central role in coordinating a comprehensive assessment of Adam's needs by a range of professionals including a pediatrician, child psychologist, and educational psychologist, and ensuring that he receives the recommended specialist therapeutic supports.

In his/her own individual work with Adam, the social worker would explain what this proposed adoptive placement might mean for him, ascertain his wishes for his future, and help him make sense of his complex life events. The social worker should commit time to meeting regularly with Adam in order to develop a trusting relationship. The social worker could use a range of play and craft activities to help Adam communicate his thoughts about significant events and relationships. For example, using buttons or dolls to create a genogram of some sort, or decorating and filling a shoe box to represent his inner reality (Winter, 2011). The social worker could seek the co-operation of birth family and previous caregivers to obtain photographs and mementos to include in a life-story book.

The social worker would complete an assessment of the teacher's suitability to adopt Adam. This evaluation would explore her experience of family relationships, and her motivation and competence to parent a child with Adam's particular needs. The social worker would acknowledge his/her dual role in both supporting and assessing the adopter and provide reassurance that admitting to difficulties would not lead to the teacher being viewed as an unsuitable parent.

Social work support would focus on helping the adopter provide the type of care-giving most likely to promote secure attachment in an adopted child, that is, being available, responding sensitively, being accepting, providing cooperative care-giving, and promoting family membership (Schofield & Beek, 2006). The adopter would be expected to avail adoption leave in order to devote time to settling Adam, and demonstrate her physical and emotional availability to meet his needs. The adopter would also be encouraged to include Adam in routines and relationships that will promote his sense of belonging as a full member of the family. The social worker would discuss with the adopter the necessity of talking with Adam about his origins to maintain his connectedness to birth family and his comfort with a dual identity.

The social worker also would help the adopter to understand the possible origin of some of Adam's difficult or puzzling behaviors to help her parent more sensitively. The social worker would give a detailed account of

Adam's family and placement history, and where possible, would arrange a meeting with previous caregivers to share information. The adopter would be encouraged to attend group training such as Adoption UK's "It's a Piece of Cake" course which is designed to help adopters understand the origin of their child's behavioral, emotional, and social difficulties in disrupted or insecure attachments.

Through regular and detailed discussion of Adam's behavior, the social worker would help the adopter to identify that the messages that he gives may not accurately communicate what he actually needs. If Adam behaves in a way that is rejecting or avoiding of care, the social worker would discuss the possibility of insecure attachment, and help the adopter respond to his underlying need for nurturance, rather than interpreting his behavior at a more superficial level (Tyrell & Dozier, 1999).

As adoptive parents empathize with the traumatized child, they are at risk of developing secondary traumatic stress disorder (Cairns, 2008). The social worker should be alert to signs of stress in the adopter and help her to maximize support from family, friends, health professionals, and peer support networks such as Adoption UK. The social worker would help the adopter to understand the transactional nature of attachment relationships (Howe & Fearnley, 2003), and identify the impact of Adam's behavior on her own responses, self-esteem, and sense of competence (Schofield & Beek, 2006).

While Adam is fostered, procedures require a multi-disciplinary review of his care. The social worker would present a recommendation on whether Adam should be adopted by his teacher. However, it would be up to a multi-disciplinary review group to agree to this care plan and for the adoption agency panel to approve the adoption placement. Following the decision to proceed with the adoption, and until the Adoption Order is made, the social worker would have a legal duty to visit regularly to monitor Adam's welfare and to support the placement. Once Adam is legally adopted, the social worker would seek to endorse his adopter's parental rights, responsibilities and autonomy, and aim to reduce his or her own input, and cease routine visiting. The social worker would re-engage with the family, at the adoptive parent's request, if assistance was needed with a specific issue at any stage in the future.

Attachment Issues among Children with Multiple Caregivers: A Social Worker from China Responds

BY AGNES LAW

Prevalence and Incidence

China has a long history of child abandonment, mostly of female children, and infanticide. This practice was widespread, spurred on by the cultural and traditional preference for male children. The motive behind abandonment was to offer the couple the opportunity to try again to have a child with a sex they preferred. Thus in several places in China, homes for abandoned children and children with unknown parentage were established to care for them (Riley, 1997; Johnson, 2002; Watson, 1975).

Other factors in child abandonment were tied to economic hardship. Though economic conditions improved in the 1980s, the Chinese government's attempt to enforce birth planning restrictions resulted in an increase in abandonment of children. To curb this, particularly in rural areas where there was much resistance to the policy, provincial governments developed policies that allowed for more than one child based on certain conditions. For instance, if a couple's first child was a girl, the wife was permitted to become pregnant again to see if they could have a boy. Also, in some places couples could have more than one child if the children were several years apart (Johnson, 2002; Zhang, 2001).

Country Policies

Adoption in China is impacted by culture and tradition. Adoption outside close bloodlines is not viewed in a positive light. Most Chinese people who adopt are more likely to adopt their own kin (Johnson, 2002). Chinese populations have many traditions and varied motivations regarding the adoption of children. Some families adopted girls for the purpose of raising them as future wives for their sons. Other families adopted boys, even when they had male children of their own, in order to have the adopted boys do the more risky chores. Some of these practices no longer exist in modern Chinese society. Though much more frequent in the past, adopting from relatives is not an uncommon practice. Such practices had economic benefits such as a guarantee that a family's estate would remain within the same extended family (Watson, 1975; Zhang, 2001; Zhang & Lee, 2011). In the adoption of males, sometimes the purpose was to perpetuate a family's heritage. In the past, adopted children were viewed as having lower social standing (Watson, 1975; Zhang & Lee, 2011).

Despite such cultural beliefs and practices, Chinese domestic adoptions exceeded international adoptions in the early 1990s until the enactment of adoption policies. Chinese government statistics on abandoned children may not be accurate. There appear to be inconsistencies in the records on child birth and adoptions as people seek to find ways to avoid government penalties. Many informal adoptions take place and many adoptive parents ignore government regulations. Thus, a lot of adopted children do not have any legal status and recognition (Riley, 1997; Zhang & Lee, 2011).

Although care services began in China as early as the 1980s in Children's Homes for orphaned and abandoned children, there was no legal protection. This situation was the case until the Interim Measures for the Administration of Foster Care was made effective on 1 January 2007 by the National Civil Affairs Bureau of the Central Government. There was, therefore, no policy covering the foster care service per se in China before that time. Children's Homes in different places had their own ways to operate so-called foster care. While some children's homes possibly started their care services earlier and might have operated in a more professional manner if they had had financial or technical support from other charities abroad, many more did not even know the concept of foster care or, in this case, alternative residential care, how to manage it, and how it could benefit orphaned and abandoned children.

Moreover, as Children's Homes in China were all under the direct management of the Civil Affairs Bureau, instead of operating for the benefit of the children, they were more administratively oriented instead of service or client oriented. In a lot of cases, orphaned and abandoned children were living in the same quarters as the elderly and the mentally retarded. As long as the children were provided with food, clothes, beds, and basic medical support, the management of the Children's Homes assumed that their responsibilities had been fulfilled, and nothing more would be provided, including medical care, education, and love.

The early days of foster care services in China benefited orphaned and abandoned children as well as rural families. Many of these families were living in poverty. Foster families received subsidies from the government, improving their living standards. This kind of foster care service provided a family-like living environment for the fostering of children. However, monitoring of the quality of foster care and assistance to the foster parents was very limited. Foster care was uncommon and communities typically received little education on the practice. They did not know how they could help, and why they should help, these children.

In the 1990s, a policy that set the legal age for adoption at 35 and also stipulated that prospective adopters should be childless, created eligibility problems for many families. The law, which was enacted in 1992, required prospective adopters to be financially sound, having the capacity to give the adopted child an education (Zhang, 2001). With restraints on the eligibility of local families, the number of children in care increased in the 1980s and early 1990s (Johnson, Banghan & Liyao, 1998; Johnson, 2002). These increases occurred at a time when the Chinese government sought to bolster its efforts in keeping its one-child birth planning policy (Zhang & Lee, 2011). This significantly affected the indigenous families who would have sought adoption through legal channels. The resulting effect was a rise in international adoptions especially from government operated centers (Johnson, 2002).

While it perhaps created an increase in the number of prospective parents by opening the adoption of Chinese children to foreigners, the law negatively impacted local adoptions. Prior to the passage of the law, many of the stipulations it contains already existed; such provisions, while less rigid, were considered to be bottlenecks to adoption. The law only made things tighter by enforcing Chinese birth control policies rather than the addressing the caregiving needs of children. The adoption law of 1991 codified existing policies that regulated adoption practices. It developed a comprehensive program to ensure that the one child per family quota was enforced (Zhang, 2001; Zhang & Lee, 2011). It also generated revenue for caregiving institutions as more foreigners adopted from the country.

A revision in the law occurred in 1999. There was a reduction in the age at which people were eligible to adopt from 35 to 30 years. This revision reflected a shift from enforcing or strengthening birth-planning regulations to addressing pertinent issues confronting childcare, such as increasing placements (Johnson, 2002). Sterilization was used as a birth control measure among those who repeatedly failed to comply with the quota. Another measure was the implementation of fines. Families who went over the quota also came under close examination (Zhang, 2001; Zhang & Lee, 2011).

The late development of social work in China is also one of the key contributing factors to the late development of foster care services in China. Before 1978, social welfare was provided under a fragmented and closed system. With recent economic developments, the demand for social services has increased. The Chinese government recently advanced a comprehensive social security policy to protect labor, the elderly, the handicapped, and children. However, the development of social services lags far behind the demand and the need for such services.

Social work as a professional discipline was first introduced in the Pearl River Delta in 1999 when one university instituted its social work degree course. There are currently fewer than 3,000 social workers working in this highly populated region. Social work has still not been professionalized in China.

A Social Worker Responds

Cases like Adam's are similar to many cases in China. When children are abandoned, the government takes on the guardian role: such children are then sent to children's homes first, before fostering can be arranged. However, sometimes children's homes do not have foster care services or no foster parents are available. It is also difficult to get the right attention and care by the social workers when their numbers are still very limited.

In practice, for about two decades in China, adoption remains controlled by the Civil Affairs Bureau. Adoption is quite a sensitive issue in the country. Local adoptions are not common due to the implementation of the one-child policy; local citizens typically choose to have their own children. Hence, most adopted children leave China for the US, Canada, Australia, or European Union countries. The Civil Affairs Bureau carefully selects children for foreign adoption who are risk free or at least whose problems are well identified and can be made known to the potential adoptive parents. Attachment disorder cases, unlike physical handicap cases, are not easily handled by the homes or government officials since they are not familiar with such problems. Attachment disorder cases are therefore treated just as serious behavioral problems. Children with such issues may not be easily selected for international adoption, which reflects the lack of social work intervention in child welfare services in China.

A recent pilot program implemented by the Civil Affairs Bureau of Guangzhou may illuminate the current situation of foster care in China. The Guangzhou Children's Welfare Institution was asked to implement a pilot program to match disabled orphans with mild physical or mental disability with foster families. Foster families would get a monthly subsidy for their services. The Guangzhou Children's Welfare Institution partnered with other social welfare agencies to hire foster couples to form a foster home in the community for up to five orphans, with social workers of the agencies also staying in the home for professional advice. However, the program was found to have a lot of problems including unclear responsibilities, lack of service procedures, and poor communication channels. Thus, it ultimately did not have any benefit for the foster children. Even in such a developed city in China, the system of foster care is still very immature, disorganized, and finance oriented. The Chinese foster care system handling cases like Adam's is clearly in its infancy.

Youth-Headed Household

BY REFILWE JEREMIAH SINKAMBA FROM BOTSWANA

Sarah is a 17-year-old girl who takes care of her two siblings, aged 10 and four years, after her parents died last year in a car accident. After the funeral, their aunt Getty, the youngest sister of Sarah's mother, volunteers to be their caregiver. She cares for four–year-old Mike, Sarah's youngest brother, and she brings food to the children each day after school. After four months, Getty tells Sarah to drop out of school and take care of Mike or else she will stop bringing them food. She says taking care of Sarah's family has become too much work for her and she needs Sarah's help. With no choice, Sarah drops out of school.

Sarah is in a romantic relationship with her classmate Ted, who comes on weekdays to help Sarah with home-studying so that she does not fall behind in her education. Additionally, studying together gives them precious time to spend in one another's company. Since she became a full time mother to Mike, Sarah has limited time for her boyfriend Ted. He feels neglected and stops coming to visit her. A few weeks later, Getty stops bringing food to the house, explaining that Sarah is old enough to handle all household duties. Sarah tries to do all the household chores including cleaning and cooking dinner for her siblings, but she is exhausted and overwhelmed. After long days of housework, Sarah drinks alcohol to put herself to sleep. She blames her parents for dying, leaving her with lots of responsibilities.

At school, Sarah's ten-year-old brother Hector does not turn in homework. He has been very quiet since his parents died and has become reserved in class. Recently, his grades have been dropping and he participates less and less in class. He is sleepy most of the time because he is scared at night, sleeping in a house without parents. At home, Hector does not talk much to his siblings. He skips dinner often. Several times Sarah has found his blankets wet when making his bed.

Recently, Getty has not been checking on the family as often as before and Sarah is running out of the money they received as benefits after their parents died. She starts to limit the amount of food she cooks. One afternoon, Sarah receives a letter of eviction from Getty's lawyer, asking them to leave the house within two weeks. Apparently, Getty has sold the property. In the midst of this turmoil, Sarah turns to an uncle for help. She tells the uncle that, after her parents died, she gave Getty, who was then their caregiver, all documents including the papers about the property. She is now surprised to be told that the house which belonged to their parents has been sold and they have to leave. After listening to Sarah, her uncle suggests he will accompany her to see a local community social worker to seek help with the housing issue, the care of her siblings, and Sarah's potential return to school.

Youth-Headed Household: A Social Worker from Hungary Responds

BY GÁBOR SZÖLLO˝SI, NIKOLETTA MÁNDI, MÁRTA ERDO˝S, JÓZSEF CSÜRKE, & JÓZSEF MADÁCSY

Prevalence and Incidence

In Hungary, orphans are not a common social problem. The absence of both parents is very rare. Although data concerning the number of Hungarian orphans is not available, numbers of orphans can be estimated from data on orphans' allowance, guardianship, and the number of clients in the child protection system. The number of people entitled for orphans allowance in 2010 was 98,519 (Social Security Statistics). A child is entitled to this allowance, if the deceased parent had acquired entitlement, which depends on the years in employment. Therefore, orphans who have one living parent are included in the above number and those orphans who are not entitled to this allowance are not represented (Central Administration of National Pension Insurance, 2010).

Another accessible source is data on guardianship. In Hungary, a minor (basically everyone under 18) is under parental control or, in the absence of such control, guardianship. Reasons for the absence of parental control vary: death of the parent(s), incapacity of the parents, judicial abolition of parental rights, or intervention by a child protection agency in cases of endangerment. In 2007 in Hungary, there were 29,407 children under guardianship. The majority of them were not orphans, but lacked parental control for other reasons.

The traditional way to care for orphans who lost both parents is appointing a guardian (without placing the child into state care); the majority of orphans are cared for by guardians. Most guardians are relatives of the child and provide care for the child in their own home. Out of the total number of children under guardianship, 6,107 were in family placements,

3,633 were with professional guardians, 6,839 were with foster parents, and 6,039 were with directors of a residential home (Institute of Social Policy and Labour, 2009).

In Hungary, there are fewer than 7,000 orphans. The majority of them are in the care of a guardian, and about 400 orphans are in the care of the state. Youth-headed households are not frequent in Hungary. Of the households in Hungary, 68.3 per cent are family-type households, 2.7 per cent are more-than-one-family or more-than-one person households. One-person households constitute 29.1 per cent, and non-family-type households make up 2.6 per cent (Hungarian Central Statistical Office, 2011). A youth-headed household qualifies as "other" in the above statistics. Data do not reveal if there are any non-family households where minors are living without adults.

Country Policies

The protection of orphans is a legal task in Hungary. The legal protection of orphans gained its modern form in the 1872 Code on Guardianship. In present-day Hungary, legal regulation is applied by the administrative authorities named the guardianship authority. Guardianship authorities—reliable bureaucratic institutions—are branches of the central government, present in every city. These authorities appoint a guardian for the orphan and decide on the case in an ex officio manner. Guardianship authorities are authorized to take measures to protect the assets of the minor.

According to legal regulations in Hungary (Act IV of 1952), minors should be under parental supervision or guardianship. Guardians are appointed and exempted by the guardianship authority; they can volunteer, but are not allowed to arbitrarily take on the role or withdraw. In most cases, guardians provide care for such children in their own households but this is not a requirement. If the child is orphaned, finding a guardian is a priority. If a guardian cannot be found (if there isn't any available relative or other person who is able and willing to fulfill the duty), other elements of the child protection system may be introduced such as adoption or state care.

Hungary has a well-developed, comprehensive child welfare and child protection system (Szollosi, 1997; Szollosi, 2004). Since the second half of nineteenth century, orphans' problems had merged into the problem of "abandoned children"; after World War II, "children-at-risk" became the all-inclusive category. The child welfare and protection system handles issues of child neglect and child maltreatment, as well as children's socio-economic, socio-cultural, and behavioral problems.

The national system of child protection came into existence in 1901, but in 1997, the Hungarian government reformed the child welfare and child protection system. New priorities included (a) the central role of children's rights, including the "best interest" principle; (b) the introduction of social work in a wide variety of cases in handling the problems of the child and the family; and (c) a new professional model in which removal from the home is the last resort. In the Hungarian system, the legal measure for orphans is permanent care. Permanent care is a legal category: the child can be placed with a foster parent, in a residential home, or in special homes for seriously ill or disabled children.

Social work in Hungary is a relatively new profession. Although social work had important theoretical and practical precedents in the first half of the twentieth century (Esztergar, 1939), it entered society only after Hungary's political transition in 1989. The transformation from a state socialist regime to a Western-type democracy was followed by broad changes in many aspects of life, including the methods of handling social problems. Clinical social work has recently been introduced in Hungary and is a less developed area within the profession. Hungarian social workers are not expected to provide therapy, only counseling: this distinction (in our view, far from being clear) refers to the "depth" of the intervention. From this perspective, therapy induces structural changes in the personality. However, Hungarian social workers do provide family therapy, a specialization of social workers.

Since 1997, social work has been an integral part of the child protection system. Social workers are not employed by the central government, but by local governments or not-for-profit organizations. The main provision for children (the "looked-after children") is social work aimed at solving the problems ("risks") of the child. This type of service is voluntary. When the child and/or the family are not willing to cooperate, the guardianship authority decides about a protective order.

When there is a serious problem in the family that endangers the children and the family is not willing to cooperate with the social worker, the children have to leave the original environment and the state provides care for them. Care provided by the state consists of legal measures and certain services at different placements. Legal measures are taking the child to emergency placement, to temporary care, or to permanent care. Recently, Hungary has tended to place children in family-like environments as much as possible; this is in contrast to historical placement of orphans in huge and often impersonal institutions.

In Hungary, nuclear families are similar to those in Western countries. Typically, only parents and their children live together in one household. During the modernization processes of Hungarian society, extended family links have loosened. However, informal support and care among close relatives is still a norm. To provide care for orphaned children is considered one of the most important family assignments. Therefore, it is probable that a guardian would be appointed from among extended family members.

A Social Worker Responds

In Hungary, Sarah and her uncle would ask for help at the local Child Welfare Service, a national social care system for children and their families. However, in a Hungarian setting, the situation would be somewhat better than in the original case. First, when the parents died, Sarah and her siblings would have automatically inherited the property. Also, a guardian would have been appointed immediately by the Guardian Authority. The guardian, Aunt Getty, would have had her activities continually monitored by the Guardian Authority to make sure that the children got the benefits to which they were entitled (e.g. orphans' allowance, family allowance), and to ensure that she used the orphans' property to serve the children's best interests. In Hungary, orphans' real estate property can be sold only with the written permission from the Guardian Authority. Aunt Getty could not obtain such permission very easily and by no means could she get it under the given circumstances. If she committed a forgery, she would be prosecuted and sentenced. Second, Sarah could not have dropped out of school as the legal school-leaving age is 18 in Hungary.

The social worker would first work to clarify the legal situation: who is the guardian? Is it Aunt Getty? If so, did she really fail to perform her guardian duties as detailed above? Did she commit a forgery? The social worker would report the case to the Guardian Authority. According to Hungarian legal regulations, Sarah cannot be expected to provide for her siblings since she herself is a child.

The best option for these children is to find a guardian within the family who can responsibly take care of the family. The second best option is adoption, and the third is state care. In the case of state care, placement with a foster parent would be the preferred solution. If neither is available, then they will receive care in a residential home. Sarah, who is very near to adulthood, could live in a student's hostel (possibly at her school) more or less independently if she so wished. The social worker would ensure that Sarah returned to school and continued her studies, as required by law.

If the uncle was appointed the new guardian and Sarah and her siblings could stay in the community, the social worker would make sure that the orphans got all the allowances and benefits to which they are entitled. These include orphans' allowances which depend on the parents' length of employment, family allowances, possibly child support, and some additional in-kind benefits such as free meals at school and kindergarten.

All the children in the case study were severely and repeatedly traumatized. For a child under 12, the loss of parents is serious issue. Therefore, all the children should receive professional help from a social worker, psychologist, or child psychiatrist, depending on their condition and on the availability of the services. Hector has already developed symptoms of anxiety. Mike was living with Aunt Getty and was turned away by her shortly after his parents died. Sarah has suffered other additional losses: after her parents died, she lost all her previous roles, her boyfriend, and the school community. Hers is an exceptionally deep identity crisis provoked by an accidental crisis.

If the social worker is trained in family therapy—this is very likely as she works in the Family Protection and Child Welfare Service—then he/she could assist in grief work and seek to restore the sibling relationships that seem to have been impaired. Therapy cannot commence until the social worker is sure that the children will stay in the local community or else he/she would add another trauma through the termination of a promising therapeutic relationship. In her therapeutic approach, the social worker would likely incorporate Ivan Boszormenyi-Nagy's contextual therapy and his theories on relational ethics (Boszormenyi-Nagy, 1987). From this theoretical perspective, Sarah is entitled to care and consideration but, in reality, suddenly lost her entitlement. This loss could result in "negative entitlement" that impairs her future relationships. Boszormenyi-Nagy's main concepts—ethics, entitlement, reciprocity, guilt, fairness, loyalty, trustworthiness within and between generations, legacy, and accountability—would play an important role in the therapy. Working through Sarah's problems, following Boszormenyi-Nagy's theoretical framework with relational ethics as the focus, would prevent further problems among the siblings and in their individual lives. In case the social worker does not have the necessary competence or time for the children's therapy, he/she would refer them to a psychotherapist or a clinical psychologist.

If the children cannot stay in the original community and instead are referred to residential care, then the social worker would help them to prepare for the new, temporary situation by guiding and informing them about their future possibilities and by transferring all the necessary information to the relevant professional. In this case, the original problem may be deepened by the trauma of transitioning into state care and the stress associated with adaptation to the new institutional environment.

Youth-Headed Household: A Social Worker from Ghana Responds

BY KWADWO OFORI-DUA

Prevalence and Incidence

Cases of youth-headed households never come to the attention of government authorities in Ghana; thus it is almost impossible to get statistics on the phenomenon. Child neglect in Ghana, however, is monitored. In the Central Region of Ghana in 2008, the Domestic Violence and Victims Support Unit (DOVVSU) of the Ghana Police Service recorded 1,131 cases of parental neglect of duty and responsibility. Many parents and guardians countrywide fail to exercise their responsibilities towards their children.

Country Policies

The Ghanaian Children's Act of 1998 (Act 560) is premised on the welfare principle that "the best interest of the child shall be paramount in any matter concerning a child" (S.2 (1)). Secondly, the Ghanaian Early Childhood and Development Policy of 2006 provides for the full protection, nurturing, and development of children with parents and their respective society.

In addition, the Legal Aid Scheme Act, 1997 (Act 542) also ensures that children are treated with utmost care in relation to their protection, growth, and development. One policy that gives practical meaning to these provisions is that of Free Compulsory Basic Education (FCUBE), which ensures that every child in Ghana receives at least six years of basic education.

These laws are enforced by state institutions. The Commission for Human Rights and Administrative Justice (CHRAJ) with a grounded mandate to investigate complaints of human rights violation resolves violation of children's rights as manifested in this case. Similarly, the Department of Social Welfare's (DSW) responsibilities include the "promotion and protection of the rights of children" (DSW, n.d, legal status and obligations, i) and "justice administration of child related issues" (DSW, n.d, legal status and obligations, ii).

A Social Worker Responds

It would be traumatic for Sarah, Hector, and Mike to lose both parents in a single day through an accident. Such calamity, if not well handled, could have a lasting and devastated effect on the children. As members of society, these children have the right to expect physical and emotional support in such a difficult situation from their guardian. Their relatives have a responsibility to exhibit love, care, and support, but they have not done so. The guardian's behavior borders on child neglect, including an attempt to deprive the children of their lawful property.

In this case, a community social worker would be an advocate who would champion the welfare of the children as stipulated by the Ghanaian Children's Act of 1998. Sarah, Hector, and Mike are all under 18 years of age and are, therefore, children in the eyes of the law. Thus, the worker will liaise with appropriate agencies such as the Ministry of Women and Children Affairs, Ghana National Commission on Children (GNCC), the Department of Social Welfare (DSW), and the Commission for Human Rights and Administrative Justice (CHRAJ) to ensure that their Aunt Getty supplies them with their basic needs as mandated by the Children's Act. The Children's Act states that "a parent or any other person who is legally liable to maintain a child or contribute towards the maintenance of the child is under a duty to supply the necessaries of health, life, education and reasonable shelter for the child" (S.47(1)).

Secondly, the community social worker would seek a court order to restrain Getty from ejecting the children from their home and from selling the house. Sections 16A and 17 (a) of the Ghanaian Intestate Succession Law 1985 (PNDCL 111) state that it is unlawful to "eject a surviving child from the matrimonial home." Clearly, Getty's action of selling the property of Sarah's parents at the expense of the children's welfare is unlawful.

Social workers are admonished by the principles of the profession to fashion intervention from the strengths perspective. Thus, a potentially useful resource here is the uncle who has shown concern for the children's situation. The worker would persuade him to take temporary custody of the children whilst he/she liaises with appropriate agencies to work out permanent maintenance strategies for the children.

The inclusion of the uncle in the solution of the case will not only provide financial support, but important psychological assistance to the young orphans. The additional help from the uncle would mean that the task of Sarah to solely care for her siblings, which makes her "exhausted and overwhelmed," will be significantly reduced. Besides, young Hector would find solace in sleeping under the protection of an adult, a psychological buffer for him against the fear of sleeping alone. He would no longer feel sleepy in class and could improve his performance.

The community worker will work with the DSW to secure day care for Mike, thus relieving Sarah so that she can concentrate on her studies. Going back to school also means that Sarah would have the opportunity to meet with her boyfriend, Ted. The reunion will significantly contribute to the emotional healing of Sarah.

In conclusion, the community social worker should act swiftly and strongly to save the children from any further negative social, economic, and psychological effects that the death of their parents would have had on them. The worker should exhibit empathy, warmth, and genuine acceptance with the goal of supporting the growth and development of the children.

Exercises

Discussion Questions

1 How do early childhood education centers and schools differ from country to country? How does this impact social workers?

2 When should government agencies step in and intervene with families? How do countries' cultural and historical contexts impact this decision?

3 What should be the definition of parental neglect? Can this be an international definition?

4 How can governments encourage communities to take more responsibility for the well-being of their children? What strategies might be effective for social workers to use in different country contexts to accomplish this?

5 What can social workers do to improve the situations of orphans in their countries?

6 Do you think governments should provide more targeted services for vulnerable children? If yes, from where should funding be accessed to do so?

7 How much monitoring of vulnerable children should governments and regulatory bodies allow? What role should social workers play in this process? How might social workers' responsibilities in this differ from country to country?

8 What mechanisms should be used to keep track of vulnerable children and their families in different country contexts? How do country and culture impact this issue?

9   What information should social workers be required to share about vulnerable children, and under what circumstances should they share this information so that ethical standards are not breached? How might this answer be different in different country contexts?

Classroom Exercises

1   Working in groups, students should create policy proposals that will improve and streamline care for vulnerable children, such as abused, neglected or orphaned children.
2   Working in groups, students should share their experiences or knowledge of the country's child welfare systems. Then discuss how social workers might intervene to improve child welfare systems in their countries.
3   Working in small groups, students create a definition of a "vulnerable child." Then discuss: the government's or society's responsibility to protect these children? What should the social worker's role be in that process?

References

Boszormenyi-Nagy, I. (1987). *Foundations of contextual therapy: Collected papers of Ivan Boszormenyi-Nagy, MD.* (pp. 20–34). New York: Brunner/Mazel.

Cairns, K. (2008). Enabling effective support: Secondary traumatic stress and adoptive families. In Hindle, D. and Shulman, G. (Eds.) (2008). *The emotional experience of adoption: A psychoanalytic perspective* (pp. 90–98).Oxon: Routledge.

"Central Administration of National Pension Insurance." (2010). Statistical Bulletin December 2010. Budapest, Hungary.

"Child Protection Act XXXI of 1997 on the protection of children and guardianship administration, Hungary." (1997). Retrieved from http://net.jogtar.hu/jr/gen/hjegy_doc.cgi?docid=99700031.TV&timeshift=1

"Children's Act, 1998 (Act 560)" [Ghana], 30 December 1998, 47 (1). Retrieved from http://www.unhcr.org/refworld/docid/44bf86454.html

Department of Health, Social Services and Public Safety (DHSSPS) (2011). "Children adopted from care in Northern Ireland 2009/10." Belfast: DHSSPS.

Department of Social Welfare (DSW) (n.d) Legal status and obligations. Retrieved from http://www.ovcghana.org/about_dsw.html

Esztergar, L. (1939). *A szocialis munka vazlata* [Elements of social work]. Pecs, Hungary: Kultura Konyvnyomda.

Ghana Laws. (1997). "Legal Aid Scheme Act 1997 (ACT 542)." Retrieved from http://ghanalegal.com/?id=3&law=166&t=ghana-laws

Howe, D., & Fearnley, S. (2003). "Disorders of attachment in adopted and fostered children: Recognition and treatment." *Clinical Child Psychology and Psychiatry*, 8, 369–87.

Hungarian Central Statistical Office (2011). Retrieved from http://www.ksh.hu/?land=en

Institute of Social Policy and Labour (2009). "Ministry of social affairs and labour: Statistical bulletin on child protection 2007." Budapest, Hungary.

Intestate Succession Law, 1985, Provisional National Defense Council (PNDC) Law 111 (PNDCL 111), Ghana (1985) 17 (a). Retrieved from http://thelandeconomist2007.synthasite.com/library/intestate-succession-law-1985-pndcl-111-

Johnson, K., Banghan, K. H., & Liyao, W. (1998). "Infant abandonment and adoption in China." *Population and Development Review*, 24, (3), 469–510.

Johnson, K. (2002). "Politics of international and domestic adoption in China." *Law and Society Review*, 36, 379–96.

Kelly, G., & McSherry, D. (2003). *Review of the Freeing Order processes in Northern Ireland*. Belfast: DHSSPS.

McSherry, D., Larkin, E., Fargas, M., Kelly, G., Robinson, C., Macdonald, G., Schubotz, D., & Kilpatrick, R. (2008). *From care to where? A care pathways and outcomes report for practitioners*. Queens University Belfast: Institute of Child Care Research.

Morris, K., & Burford, G. (2007). "Working with children's existing networks-building better opportunities." *Social Policy and Society*, 6, (2), 209–17.

New Zealand Ministry of Health (2010). UNGASS country progress report New Zealand: Reporting Period: January 2008–December 2009. Retrieved from http://www.moh.govt.nz/moh.nsf/pagesmh/7565/$File/UNGASS-country-progress.

New Zealand Government (2011). "The green paper for vulnerable children: Every child thrives, belongs, achieves." Retrieved from http://www.children-sactionplan.govt.nz/

Northern Ireland Assembly (2010). "Overview of adoption: research and library service briefing paper 126/10." Belfast: NIA.

Northern Ireland Factsheets (NIA) (2010) Retrieved from http://www.medical-protection.org/uk/northern-ireland-factsheets

O'Halloran, K. J. (2001). "Adoption in the two jurisdictions of Ireland: A case study of changes in the balance between public and private law." *International Family Law Journal*, 43, 1–16.

Riley, N. E. (1997). "American adoptions of Chinese girls: The socio-political matrices of individual decisions." *Women's Studies International Forum*, 20, (1), 87–102.

Rushton, A., & Dance, C. (2004). "The outcomes of late permanent placements: the adolescent years." *Adoption and Fostering*, 28, (1), 49–58.

Rushton, A., Monck, E., Upright, H., & Davidson, M. (2006). "Enhancing adoptive parenting: devising promising interventions." *Child and Adolescent Mental Health*, 11, (1), 25–31.

Schofield, G., & Beek, M. (2006). *Attachment handbook for foster care and adoption*. London: BAAF.

Simmonds, J. (2008). "Developing a curiosity about adoption: A psychoanalytic perspective." In D. Hindle & G. Shulman (Eds) (2008). *The emotional experience of adoption a psychoanalytic perspective* (pp. 27–41). Oxon: Routledge.

Szollosi, G. (Ed.) (2004). *Gyermekjoleti alapellatas. Segedanyag a szocialis szakvizsgahoz.* [Basic child welfare services. Textbook for professional social examination]. Budapest: NCSSZI.

Szollosi, G. (1997). "Protection of the family by family law and other instruments." In L. Salgo (Ed.). *The family justice system. Past and future, experiences and propects. Collegium Workshop Series No. 3* (pp. 81–109). Budapest: Collegium Budapest, Institute for Advanced Study,

Triseliotis, J., Feast, J., & Kyle, F. (2005). *The adoption triangle revisited: A study of adoption, search and reunion experiences*. London: BAAF.

Tyrell, C., & Dozier, M. (1999). "Foster parents' understanding of childrens' problematic behavior strategies." *Adoption Quarterly, 2*, 49–64.

UNICEF CEECIS (n.d.). Central and Eastern European Commonwealth of Independent States. Retrieved from http://www.unicef.org/ceecis/

UNICEF (2011). Opportunity in Criss: Preventing HIV from early adolescence to early adulthood. Retrieved from http://www.unicef.org/aids/index_58689.html

Watson, J. (1975). "Agnates and outsiders: Adoption in a Chinese lineage." *Man, 10*, 293–306.

Winter, K. (2011). *Building relationships and communicating with young children: A practical guide for social workers*. Oxon: Routledge.

Zhang, W. (2001). "Institutional reforms, population policy, and adoption of children: Some observations in a North China village." *Journal of Comparative Family Studies, 32* (2), 303–18.

Zhang, Y., & Lee, G. R (2011). "Parents' motivations and preferences in adoption intercountry versus transracial adoption: Analysis of adoptive." *Journal of Family Issues, 32*, 75–98.

8 Adolescents

By Joanna E. Bettmann

The number of adolescents in the world is increasing. In 2009, the United Nations estimated that there were 1.2 billion adolescents in the world, comprising 18 per cent of the world's population (UNICEF, 2011). Adolescents are a significant percentage of the world's population and a population with whom social workers often engage. This chapter on adolescents covers the topics of adolescents committing crimes, gay adolescents coming out, and teenage pregnancy. These are all common cases in which social workers encounter this age group.

Case study #1

An Adolescent Committing Crime

BY ELIOT SYKES AND MARK EDWARD BARR FROM THE US

Hunter is a 12-year-old boy. He is the youngest of three children: he has a brother who is 17 and a sister, aged 15. Hunter was raised in a lower middle-class area at the edge of a city. His parents divorced two years ago. His father had long been physically abusive to his mother. Hunter now lives with his mother, sister, and grandparents in a community about four hours away from his home. His mother brought Hunter and his sister to live with her parents when the divorce occurred. His older brother decided to live with their father and to stay in their home.

Hunter's mom has just recently started to date other men and is spending more time with one boyfriend in particular. The grandparents are helping her raise the kids and they babysit often.

Hunter has been enrolled in a new school and is adjusting to making new friends. Recently, he was caught stealing pants from a department store and he was caught spray-painting graffiti on a building last month. Hunter appears to be frustrated with fitting-in at school, with his friends and adjusting to the new life. Hunter is brought into a social worker's office by his grandmother, who is worried about him.

An Adolescent Committing Crime: A Social Worker from the Pacific Islands Responds

BY ROBIN L. DAVIS

Prevalence and Incidence

Hawaii is the most ethnically diverse state in the US (Frankfort-Nachmias & Leon-Guerrero, 1997). In this mix, recent immigrants as well as the descendants of the island's original inhabitants are among the most dispossessed; consequently, youth actively involved in gangs are drawn predominantly from groups that have recently immigrated to the state (Samoans and Filipinos) or from the increasingly marginalized Native Hawaiian population. Most girls (90 per cent) and boys (80 per cent) have a family member who belonged to a gang (Joe & Chesney-Lind, 1995). Like other major cities, Hawaii's capital city of Honolulu has witnessed a rapid growth in gang activity and gang membership. In 1988, the Honolulu police estimated that there were 22 gangs with 450 members. In 1991, the number of gangs climbed to 45 with an estimated membership of 1,020. By 1993, the number of gangs reached 171 with 1,267 members (Chesney-Lind et al. 2003).

Pacific Islander youth suffer other stressors as well. The process of living in a traditional Pacific Islander household and at the same time living in an Americanized community, trying to align with a new environment and educational system, adds both emotional and physical stress that hinders healthy development among some youth (Vakalahi, 2009). Another stressor youth face is racism from teachers and school officials. Some teachers and administrators perceive Pacific Islander students as trouble makers and not as intelligent. Others stereotype them as athletes, rather than students, due to their large stature.

Country Policies

When Samoan children are caught between different value systems, and as the village system of social controls weakens, the pressures and problems in Samoan families multiply. In Samoan communities, locals rely on the open community structure to provide community awareness of youth behavior and consequentially to deter antisocial acts and to ensure conformity. The public pronouncement of crime, punishment, and village gossip are powerful instruments for social control and social conformity. This method of social control appears to be particularly important to adolescents who, by virtue of school and school activities, are able to escape the control of their parents and relatives. Public pressures for conformity to ideal behavior patterns weaken substantially with urban living (Janes, 1990). Crime control in Samoa is primarily generated by the community, which relies on social expectations and norms. Samoan youth who migrate from Samoa to the mainland US may perceive fewer social consequences as they transition from a more rural, community environment to urban communities where legal consequences are primarily enforced by law enforcement (Davis, 2005).

This difference in social control may result in Samoan youth entering into the juvenile justice system at higher rates than other ethnic groups. When American and Western Samoans come to the US, not only are there more options for gaining access to controlled substances and getting involved in risky behaviors, e.g., drugs, gangs, and weapons, but also fewer eyes are watching over them as part of their community not only to keep them in check, but also to help them develop in a prosocial manner.

A Social Worker Responds

The Samoan self has been described as having meaning only in relationship with other people, not as an individual. This self could not be separated from the "va" or relational space that occurs between an individual and parents, siblings, grandparents, aunts, uncles, and other extended family and community members. In providing mental health services, it is important to include the context, or relationship between family and community, since the "va" is an important source of meaning and life support in the process of healing. For Hunter, family counseling, and inclusion of some elements reflecting on the relationship between him and his family, his old neighborhood, community, and culture would be important for healing and reconnecting with a positive sense of self identity.

In the working phase of this case, the social worker must perform an assessment and then identify several treatment goals with the input of

Hunter and his primary support system, which is his grandmother. It is important to include family members as healing, in the context of Samoan individuals, happens within the family. After covering confidentiality with each family member, the social worker should inquire what each person would like to gain from his/her interactions in attending counseling.

One of the most important steps in working with Pacific Islander families is "joining," creating a therapeutic alliance with the entire family, as well as the identified client. Many Pacific Islanders are new to the therapy process. It is important to be respectful and polite, and to explain the role of the social worker, while building a relationship with the family. According to Lee (2002), "Appropriate self-disclosure may facilitate positive cultural alliance and an increased level of trust and confidence. Asking nonthreatening personal questions can put the family at ease. It is also important to avoid direct confrontation, to demand greater emotional disclosure, or to discuss culturally taboo subjects such as sex or death" (p. 44).

The social worker should focus on the immediate crisis or problem that brought the family to the agency, in this case Hunter's delinquency. Usually, families seek counseling for one member's actions and are unaware of their own contributing behavior. They might not want to discuss their contribution to the problem in front of the children. In Samoan culture, respect for parents is always expected.

For Pacific Islander populations, most problems are handled within the parameters of the family or extended family. Therefore, families may be ashamed to see a social worker. The social worker can help reframe this embarrassment by ensuring the family of confidentiality, empathizing with uncomfortable feelings, and praising family members for their willingness to support an identified client within a family system. In the case of Hunter, it would be important to normalize any shame around his delinquent behavior. It is also important to instill hope for both him and his grandmother with an indication that Hunter can move past this phase and go on to learn from his flaws and live a prosocial life.

Many Asian and Pacific Islander clients come to their first session believing that the clinician is an authority who can tell them what is wrong and how to solve their problems. It is helpful for the clinician to establish credibility right away to ensure that the client will return. An air of confidence, empathic understanding, maturity, and professionalism are all-important ingredients. However, it is critical to balance client-self determination and respect for the client with providing a safe environment of expertise for the client system. Since Pacific Islander clients often do not return for a second session, it would be critically important to instill hope and confidence in both Hunter and his grandmother so that they could work with the social worker to overcome Hunter's issues.

One of the functions of therapy is to mobilize the family's cultural strengths. Strengths in Pacific Islander families may include support from the extended family, a strong sense of obligation and family loyalty, parental sacrifice for the children's future, filial piety, strong focus on educational achievement and the work ethic, and support from the ethnic community. In many circumstances, especially when family members are coping with death, loss, or unpredictable changes, discussions of religious stories or philosophical teachings from native cultures can be very therapeutic.

In addition to determining a Samoan family's primary language, a social worker must work to understand the family's communication style. Pacific Islander Americans are traditionally taught to employ indirect styles of communication and to avoid direct confrontation. Negative emotions such as anger, grief, and depression may be expressed indirectly. Even positive feelings such as love are frequently not expressed in an open manner. The social worker may have to draw out the meanings of major issues and emotions, as well as be careful not to come across as too direct or pushy. The social worker will most likely have to draw out Hunter's thoughts and emotions as he likely will not want to communicate much.

Both the family and community become active participants in the process of change and are key elements to the change process (Browne & Mills, 2001). Context is a key concept in work with Pacific Islanders, and reflects the importance of families and communities taking responsibility for the direction of mental health services. This strategy will be enhanced if social workers continually engage themselves in self-awareness activities, serving to examine their own attitudes toward racism, oppression, cultural diversity, and identity (Mokuau, 1991).

An Adolescent Committing Crime: A Social Worker from the US Responds

BY ROB BUTTERS

Prevalence and Incidence

Juveniles accounted for 16 per cent of all violent crime and 26 per cent of all property crime in the US in 2008. Juvenile crime in the US has been steadily declining since its peak in 1994. The most common crimes committed by juveniles are property crimes like vandalism, robbery, burglary, or theft. Juveniles account for nearly half of all arson, 18 per cent of sexual assaults, and about 10 per cent of murders. Females make up 30 per cent of juvenile offenders and ethnic minorities, especially African Americans, are disproportionally represented throughout the juvenile justice system (Puzzanchera, 2009). These statistics show that juvenile crime is a significant social problem both in terms of costs to society and the development of a dangerous criminal trajectory for these young boys and girls.

Country Policies

The US provides social services to at-risk and delinquent youth through a myriad of social service programs, administered both publically and privately. Youth may be referred to the attention of a social worker through several channels: by family members, as in Hunter's case; by schools; by community-based prevention programs; or by the juvenile court system. The US established its first juvenile court in Chicago, Illinois in 1899. Today, there are juvenile courts throughout the country. These courts operate less formally than adult criminal courts and are based on the philosophy that youth are less culpable for their offenses and are more amenable to treatment and rehabilitation. Most youth are eligible for adjudication in juvenile court until age 18, but this varies by jurisdiction and nature of the offense.

Most youth adjudicated in the juvenile courts face sanctions such as fines, community service, house arrest, or supervision by juvenile probation. Fines may range from US $25 for simple court processing fees to mandatory fees of several hundreds or even thousands of dollars. Community service hours are ordered in nearly all juvenile cases, reflecting a value that service to the community can play a role in rehabilitation. It is also required for the juvenile to repay the costs of crime to the community. Most community service is completed at a non-profit organization or government entity, or can be simply picking up trash along a highway or at a city park. House arrest is a common sanction in which a juvenile is confined to his/her home and only allowed to leave for sanctioned activities like school or church. Most juveniles will be sentenced to house arrest for one to two weeks following disposition as both a consequence and to incapacitate the youth so that he/she desists from further offending. Juvenile probation is community supervision that requires the juvenile to meet regularly with a probation officer, restrictions on activities outside the home, early curfews, and submitting to drug testing and/or searches of their residence or person. The juvenile courts often refer youth to counseling or instruct them to be temporarily removed from their homes for placement in a community-based, residential treatment program. More serious offenders may be placed in secure treatment facilities, such as prisons, to ensure their own safety and the safety of the community.

In providing case management services, assessments, and mental health treatment, social workers make up a large proportion of the service providers for these juvenile offender populations. The most serious and dangerous youth criminal offenders are often transferred to the adult criminal system where they are adjudicated and sentenced as adults. Until a recent 2005 Supreme Court ruling, US juveniles could be executed for crimes committed prior to their eighteenth birthday. Now the maximum penalty for a juvenile who is transferred to adult court is life in prison.

Social work in the US continues to evolve as a profession, continually redefining the parameters of practice, roles and responsibilities, and ethics. Social workers continue to advocate for oppressed and disadvantaged populations and strive to promote social and economic justice. Social workers are employed in many different capacities in the juvenile justice system. Bachelor's degree-trained social workers function as probation officers or case managers, while Master's trained social workers may provide mental health therapy or assessment services and are required to be licensed as a clinical social worker. Social workers are licensed at both the Bachelor's and Master's levels by completing a degree in social work, passing a board exam, and doing internships under the supervision of a licensed social worker.

Social workers now have numerous evidence-based interventions and research-based theoretical models that can be used to effectively and efficiently respond to crime and delinquency. As recently as the 1970s, most people thought that "nothing works" in deterring crime and treating criminal offenders because there was a lack of solid empirical research on crime and delinquency (Martinson, 1974). Fortunately over the last 40 years, we have accumulated a substantial body of literature that provides clear evidence that certain programs do work and that we can reduce and prevent most juvenile crime. The Risk-Need-Responsivity (Andrews & Bonta, 2010) and Restorative Justice (Unbreit & Armour, 2010) models are ubiquitous in programs for youth in the US and these models will be used as a framework to respond to Hunter in this case analysis.

A Social Worker Responds

Hunter has been brought to see a clinical social worker by his grandmother because she is concerned about his adjustment to his new school and his recent criminal activity. A US social worker in this case would orient Hunter and his grandmother to the treatment process and conduct a biopsychosocial assessment of Hunter across a variety of life domains. This assessment would yield a diagnostic profile and possibly a mental health diagnosis. This diagnosis is important to pursue funding for treatment from insurance or third-party payers. Unfortunately funding for treatment, even treatment for a significant medical or mental health disorder, is not guaranteed in the US

The assessment would conclude with the social worker providing recommendations for treatment based on the presenting problem, history, and mental health diagnosis. Based on the assessment, the social worker would develop measurable treatment goals and then contract with Hunter and his grandmother about further services.

Based on Hunter's presenting problems, the most urgent issues appear to be his escalating criminal behaviors, his adjustment to a new school, and his disrupted family relationships. Hunter does not appear to have a long history of criminal or behavior problems. Based on his young age and lack of other significant mental health problems, the interventions will target the risk factors in his immediate environment (Andrews & Bonta, 2010) through short-term, solution-focused therapy (Nelson & Thomas, 2009). In addition, social work intervention with Hunter will focus on resolving the harm done to the victims of his criminal activity through victim-offender mediation (Umbreit & Armour, 2010).

According to the Risk-Need-Responsivity model (Andrews & Bonta, 2010), there are three principles that should be considered when treating criminal offenders. The Risk principle states that the intensity of the intervention should be based on the risk for future offending, with low risk offenders receiving little or no intervention while high risk offenders receive intensive services. Hunter appears to be a low to moderate risk for reoffending so his treatment will be targeted and short-term. The Need principle states that treatment should target specific criminogenic needs, meaning specific factors demonstrated through research to reduce recidivism or future offending. Hunter's treatment will target the most salient risk factors that could contribute to future delinquency: his criminal behaviors, parenting, adjustment to divorce, family structure, and school bonding (Wasserman et al., 2003). The Responsivity principle states that interventions should be based on the offender's individual characteristics like culture, learning style, and ability. Hunter is an adolescent and his treatment must be tailored to his unique developmental needs, his personality, and his family.

The first step a social worker would take with this adolescent client is to engage the youth in treatment by creating a strong therapeutic alliance. This action would be accomplished by first meeting with Hunter and his grandmother to gather important background and family information, then meeting with Hunter alone. US adolescents have a developmentally-appropriate need to be seen as independent and to be respected as unique people. It is important for the social worker to establish rapport with Hunter so that he perceives the social worker as his advocate. Exploring Hunter's perception of the problems in his life and his strengths will help his treatment as well as build rapport.

Engaging the rest of Hunter's family will facilitate short-term family therapy to address his estrangement from his father and older brother, his feelings about his mother's boyfriend, and his feelings about his parent's divorce. With Hunter and the grandmother's permission, the social worker would place a call to the mother and father to gather additional information about Hunter and invite them to family therapy. Based on the severity of the domestic violence and the level of conflict between the parents, family therapy may be conducted with the whole family or with sub-groups within the family. Family therapy would address issues related to communication, conflict resolution, roles and boundaries in the family, consistency in consequences and discipline, and rewards for positive behaviors.

Hunter's school adjustment and bonding to his new school is an important risk factor that should be addressed in treatment. Hunter's feelings about changing schools and making new friends should be discussed in individual treatment sessions. During these sessions, the social worker could brainstorm with Hunter about ways he has made friends in the past and identify opportunities at his new school or community and friendships with positive peers. Activities like school clubs, athletic teams, community centers, scouting, or church organizations would be places he could meet friends. Additionally, the social worker could do outreach to a school counselor or teacher to make them aware of Hunter's struggles.

Hunter's criminal activity, his theft and graffiti, would not likely warrant an overly strong response from the criminal justice system. He would probably be cited by law enforcement and ordered to appear before a judge or commissioner. Most juvenile cases do not go to trial because they are resolved through plea bargaining. Plea bargaining is when an offender admits to the crime in exchange for dropping other charges or for a reduced sentence. The most likely disposition in crimes like his would be an order to complete community service. The principles of restorative justice would prescribe that Hunter should work to repair the harm from his behavior so he could be ordered to paint over graffiti in his neighborhood.

The social worker could advocate for Hunter in court by attending the court hearings and formulating a plan with the family to complete his community service. Most juvenile courts subscribe to the Balanced and Restorative Justice Model (Umbreit & Armour, 2010) that seeks to balance the needs of community safety, accountability, and the need for rehabilitation. In Hunter's case, the social worker could facilitate victim-offender mediation meetings in which Hunter would take responsibility and apologize to the manager of the store from which he stole the pants, and to the owner of the building where he painted the graffiti. During this mediation, Hunter, the victims and those affected by his behavior would agree on a plan for him to repair the harm he has caused and to make restitution to them. This plan can be completed through some form of service to the victims. Victim offender mediation can be a very powerful intervention and meets not just Hunter's needs, but the needs of the community as well.

Treatment would likely last between 60 and 90 days and would terminate when the treatment goals are resolved and Hunter is functioning well at school, in the community, and within his family. The most intensive treatment would take place toward the beginning of treatment, tapering off toward the end as risk factors are addressed and resolved.

Case study #2

A Gay Adolescent Coming Out

BY JEANNA JACOBSEN FROM THE US

Lydia was a 16-year-old girl who lived with her parents and sisters in a rural community. Recently, she had begun having sexual thoughts about her best friend. These feelings were new. She had had close friendships with other girls in the past, but this time was different. Her friendship with her best friend had gotten closer over the past few months. They spent all their time together and told each other everything. They were always hugging or touching each other in some way. She thought that all girls had similar relationships. But the other day when expressing these thoughts, her best friend kissed her and said, "I love you, too." She had not known how to respond. She did know that the feelings that she had in that moment were stronger and more intense then she had ever experienced.

Now she felt confused. She never understood why all the other girls her age focused so much attention on boys. She would rather play games with the boys than think of them romantically. She just assumed that someday she would get married the way women did. She had so many questions. What did these current thoughts mean about who she was? Could it be that it was just this specific girl that she loved? Was this just a phase?

One of her classmates had "come out" as gay about a year ago. Everyone knew that he had sex with other men. Some of the kids made fun of him and called him names. She did not know how he dealt with that. He said once that he recognized his sexuality as a very young child and he did not want to hide anymore. Lydia did not feel as certain. She knew that he belonged to a group that advocated for homosexual people. She felt afraid that if she talked to him about the group, someone might find out and then her peers would ostracize her. Society treated girls differently when it came to sex.

She thought about her family. She remembered hearing some of her family members making disparaging remarks about homosexuals. She felt afraid of how they would react if they knew about her feelings; she did not want to disappoint them. She had heard of some families rejecting and disowning their children who came out as gay. She did not want to lose her family. She did not know who she could talk to about this. She wondered if she should just ignore these feelings. She began feeling depressed thinking that something must be wrong with her. She decided to see a social worker to talk about her feelings and worries.

A Gay Adolescent Coming Out: A Social Worker from Ghana Responds

BY KWADWO OFORI-DUA

Prevalence and Incidence in Ghana

Until 2006, many Ghanaians assumed that homosexuality did not exist in Ghana. However, with Ghanaian media reportage in 2006 about the convening of gays and lesbians for an international conference in Ghana, there was a huge public outcry and widespread condemnation. This ignited debates about homosexuality all over the nation (Luckie, n.d). Homosexuality may be pervasive in Ghana, but appears notably in Takoradi in the Western Region, the capital city Accra, and other large cities like Kumasi and Tema (Attipoe, 2004; Thoreson & Cook, 2011).

Same-gender sexual relations generally run counter to the sociocultural beliefs and values in Ghana. There are no registered Lesbian, Gay, Bisexual, and Transgender (LGBT) organizations in the country. Discrimination against members of the LGBT community is widespread. There is an apparent lack of support for gays from the police. Attempts at extorting money and the blackmailing of gays are common experiences gay men face. Further, gay men in prisons are often victims of abuse (Attipoe, 2004; Thoreson & Cook, 2011).

Country Policies

The issue of homosexuality gained prominence in Ghana in September, 2006 when a proposed LGBT rights conference was scheduled to take place at the Accra International Conference Centre; it was subsequently banned by the government (Ghana, n.d). The Minister of State at the Information Ministry stated the government's position when he said, "Government would like to make it absolutely clear that it shall not permit the proposed conference anywhere in Ghana. Unnatural carnal knowledge is illegal under our criminal code. Homosexuality, lesbianism and bestiality are therefore offences under the laws of Ghana" (Luckie, n.d, Conference Causes Unrest section, para. 3). He added that "the government does not condone any such activity which violently offends the culture, morality and heritage of the entire people of Ghana. Supporting such a conference, or even allowing it, will encourage that tendency which the law forbids" (Luckie, n.d, Conference Causes Unrest section, para. 4).

Homosexuality is a criminal offense in Ghana. However, the criminal code (1960) does not specifically define homosexuality as illegal. The criminal code (1960) lists the following: "Whoever has unnatural carnal knowledge— (a) of any person of the age of sixteen years or over without his consent shall be guilty of a first degree felony...; or (b) of any person of sixteen years or over with his consent is guilty of a misdemeanor;.... (2) Unnatural carnal knowledge is sexual intercourse with a person in an unnatural manner or with an animal" (S. 104). Ghana's criminal code clearly (judges) classifies homosexuality as a sexual offense comparable to bestiality, assault, and rape in the criminal code. In Ghana, there is no legal recognition of same-sex couples and the laws that prohibit homosexuality affirm the cultural and religious orientation of the country.

Prior to the 1900s, the management of social problems in Ghana remained the sole responsibility of individual families. However, following the industrial revolution in Europe in the early 1900s and its concomitant demands for new raw materials from African countries, men and women left their villages for work, thereby losing the support and control of their families. In the urban centers where they settled, they lost the security and sense of belonging they had enjoyed in their villages. As a result of this new social structure, parents had little or no time to spend with their children. Thus, various social problems emerged, such as truancy, parental neglect, marital dissolution, family dysfunction, and juvenile delinquency. The Ghanaian government introduced social services to address these social problems around 1946 (Lord Beveridge Report, 1944). Today, state-provided social services include community care, child rights and protection, care for the aged, and social justice administration among others (Opoku, 1991).

In Ghana, social workers perform a range of functions in a variety of settings. In hospital settings, social workers form part of the medical team, assisting patients who have personal problems such as the maintenance of their houses/homes, job security, and other domestic problems while on admission (DSW Records, 2011). Social workers are also found working in Ghanaian prisons and correctional centers, acting as liaison officers between the prison authorities and the families of the inmates, as well as providing assistance to inmates in preparing documents to appeal against their sentences, providing clothes during their incarceration and transportation to their designations when discharged (DSW Records, 2011). Many Ghanaian social workers also work in child welfare domains, providing care and protection to children in child welfare institutions such as children's homes, orphanages, and day care centers. Other workers also act as advocates, speaking for and on behalf of children who are likely to be abused, sold into slavery, or forced into child labor. Ghanaian social workers work with the aged and infirm, linking them to resources which can provide food, clothing, shelter, and medical treatment (DSW Records, 2011). A number of NGOs utilize the services of social workers in their development projects. For instance, the Christian Council of Ghana has three professional social workers on its staff at the Budumburam Refugee Centre in the Central region where Liberia refugees are camped.

Social workers in Ghana also help resolve domestic conflicts and problems, roles which in the past were the preserve of the extended family and lineage system. For instance, the Domestic Violence and Victims Support Unit (DOVVSU) of the Ghana Police Service at times utilizes the services of social workers in resolving family and marriage problems. Through this technique, many domestic issues are settled out of court.

Social work is growing in Ghana. The School of Social Work in Accra has been offering Bachelors-level diploma training in social work since 1946, but now the profession is gaining ground with the introduction of under-graduate and graduate courses in Ghanaian public universities. Even with these programs, social work has not gained recognition as in countries like the US and UK.

A Social Worker Responds

The case study gives a picture of a confused adolescent struggling to understand a new sexual feeling she has developed for her best friend. It suggests the client's inner confusion, turmoil, and stress resulting from being forced by society to hide her feelings and live in fear of being shamed or rejected. Lydia may also be experiencing some depression and indecision.

The social worker's first response should be to allay the fears of homophobia expressed by Lydia. The client is in a state of confusion and emotional discomfort because of the fear of being discriminated against and ostracized, the fear of losing her family and loved ones, and the desire to protect her family against societal neglect and embarrassment. The social worker would allay the fears of the client by first demonstrating a high level of empathy and acceptance through explaining and revealing that he/she understands her situation. The worker would then educate her on the development and changes associated with transition from childhood to adolescent. The purpose of this exercise would be to assure her that what she is experiencing is a normal feeling to any growing child. What makes her situation different or problematic is her affection or attraction to the same sex. Such assurance would likely bring relief to Lydia.

After allaying her fears, the social worker would then proceed to prepare a social history and assessment report for the benefit of other professionals who may be involved in the management of Lydia's case. The social history and assessment report would enable the worker and other professionals to get a deeper understanding of the client and her social environment (the family, community, and school) and how these interact to affect the problem at hand.

In preparing the social history and assessment report, the social worker would first interview Lydia. He/she would corroborate information obtained from the client by visiting her family, neighborhood, school etc. if necessary to observe things for him/herself. This action would enable the worker to create an intervention strategy or make the necessary recommendations for addressing the client's problem. The worker would also schedule an interview with the client's best friend to collect the necessary information about her, her family, and her environment. This information would enable the worker to know the root cause of the client's problem, more especially the extent to which Lydia's situation is influenced by her best friend.

For a social worker in Ghana, the main focus is to prevent Lydia from embracing homosexuality as it is socially frowned upon. Since Lydia's problem is reflected in her thoughts and emotions, counseling would be the most appropriate strategy to help her. The social worker would solicit the services of other specialists as needed. For example, to see if Lydia is of sound mind and able to concentrate on her studies, the social worker might arrange for her to see a psychologist who will counsel her to be in the right frame of mind. An educational counselor would assess her performance in school and offer advice and techniques that would help her to focus on her education and take her mind off the sexual thoughts, change her thoughts about herself, and also help her to deal with her new experience.

The social worker could also seek the services of a religious leader to help Lydia deal with the emotional aspects of the problem. Ghana is largely a religious nation: almost every Ghanaian belongs to a religious group. The social worker could involve a religious leader in the counseling of Lydia. Many Ghanaians are more willing to open up and confide in their pastors, Imams, and other religious leaders than other professionals. If Lydia falls within this category, then referral to her religious leader would be very useful.

The social worker should also elicit the support of Lydia's parents. The parents should provide emotional support, encouraging her to eradicate all the negative thoughts about herself. The social worker, in conjunction with her parents, should offer love and guidance since Lydia is not mature enough to discern right from wrong.

Because the devil finds jobs for idle hands, the social worker should ensure that Lydia gets involved in an activity that is productive or recreation that would take her mind off her sexual thoughts. The worker should also ensure that she associates with people who can help her overcome the problem. For example, if she is religious, she should be encouraged to associate more with her Christian brothers and sisters. Through fellowship and interaction with others, Lydia would be relieved from her anxieties and distress.

The social worker's role here is to coordinate the activities of all the other professionals involved in Lydia's case. The worker would also have to monitor her progress in school, social interactions, group association, religious activities, and her general well-being. It would be incumbent on the worker to liaise with her family and school to ensure that the client does not lack anything that is important to her well-being and welfare.

A Ghanaian social worker should advise and not impose anything on clients contrary to their choices. However, the cultural context of Lydia's case would prevent the client from making a choice in this case. Since homosexuality is illegal in Ghana, the cultural, moral, and legal values of Ghana would considerably affect the social work intervention in this case.

A Gay Adolescent Coming Out: A Social Worker from the US Responds

BY J. MATT UPTON

Prevalence and Incidence

Research indicates that about 3.5 per cent of the US population identifies as gay, lesbian, or bisexual, with about 0.03 per cent of the population identifying as transgendered. Among American adolescents, approximately 5 per cent identify as gay, lesbian, or bisexual (Bagley & Tremblay, 2000).

Country Policies

The LGBT human rights movement currently underway in the US (Adiatu, 2009) continues to struggle for LGBT people to have the right to marry, freedom from discrimination in the workplace, and protection from violent hate crimes. US federal policy permits same-sex relationships, but does not allow same-sex marriage. However, several states have modified their state laws to permit same-sex marriages, i.e. New York, Vermont, New Hampshire, Massachusetts, Iowa, and Connecticut.

However, LGBT youth face a difficult climate in the US, because they are more likely to be verbally and physically abused by peers and family members than heterosexual youth. They are also more likely to participate in criminal activity, substance abuse, and prostitution (Savin-Williams, 1994). LGBT adolescents are two to three times more likely to attempt suicide than their heterosexual peers (Nelson, 1994). Notably, among homeless adolescents, 25 to 40 per cent are LGBT (Nelson, 1994).

In 1973, the American Psychological Association (APA) voted not to identify homosexuality as a mental illness, removing it from the Diagnostic and Statistical Manual (Morgan & Nerison, 1993). More recently, the APA stated, "Same-sex sexual attractions, behavior and orientations per se are normal and positive variants of human sexuality—in other words, they do not indicate either mental or developmental disorders" (APA, 2009). All of the major US mental health professional organizations agree that homosexuality is not a mental illness.

A Social Worker Responds

The role of Lydia's social worker is to support Lydia and foster her self-esteem in discovering her sexual identity so that she may lead a full and productive life. When Lydia enters the office, the first step for the social worker is to introduce him/herself to Lydia and make sure she feels safe in the office environment using non-judgmental language. The therapist will listen closely to her story, and help her look at her sexual identity in more depth. In this session, the social worker may want to talk to Lydia about her internalized homophobia. If she has the experience that her family does not approve of same-sex attraction, she may also hold some of these beliefs to be true, thus creating a very large obstacle to her accepting her own sexuality. Other considerations for Lydia in her coming-out process include her community's views on same-sex attraction. Is she a member of a religious institution that views homosexuality unfavorably? How does she view herself and her evolving view of her sexuality within the context of these communities? How can she reconcile these identities with her possible new identity within the LGBT community?

The coming-out experience for people who identify as LGBT can be empowering. Lydia still questions her sexuality at this point so, though it is appropriate to discuss this process with her, it is important to let her know that there is no rush for her to open up to her friends and family about her same-sex attraction. She needs to experience this process at her own pace. If Lydia decides that she is comfortable coming out, the social worker needs to work with her to identify people in her life in whom she feels she can confide. Can she confide in one of her parents, sisters, or her whole family unit? Would she feel better talking about this with another relative, perhaps an aunt, uncle, or cousin? She may want to start with a close friend whom she trusts so that she can become comfortable with discussing her sexual orientation with someone she cares about and who cares about her.

Once Lydia has identified someone she would like to confide in about her sexuality, the social worker may use role play as a method to help Lydia work through the coming-out process. In the role play, Lydia would play herself and the social worker would take the role of the person to whom Lydia would like to come out. Through this process, Lydia can practice saying the words out loud. The social worker may present through role plays what it would be like for Lydia to experience an unfavorable reaction to her confession of same-sex attraction. This practice will give Lydia an opportunity to see how she might deal with this sort of reaction before she has to experience it in real life. The social worker may also want to switch roles, allowing Lydia to take the role of the friend or family member so that the social worker can model some ways Lydia could approach the topic.

As Lydia prepares to come out to her family, it may be helpful for her to solicit support from the LGBT community. A social worker who is LGBT affirmative, meaning a practitioner who is a supportive advocate for his/her LGBT clients, in any community should have access to information regarding organizations where Lydia might feel safe to connect with others who are going through similar experiences. Joining these organizations, such as a local LGBT Center, which often offers an array of support groups and drop in facilities for individuals who identify as LGBT, will give Lydia the opportunity to see how others have answered these questions for themselves as well as providing her with a sense of connection which may help her manage frustrations and disappointments she might encounter in the coming-out process.

Groups for LGBT adolescents also stress the importance of personal safety. Teens who feel isolated are more likely to participate in dangerous activities such as substance abuse and unprotected sex. Encouraging Lydia to engage with a supportive community organization may provide an opportunity for her to educate herself about how to safely explore her sexual identity. Finally, as the social worker gets to know Lydia, he/she may want to pay attention to her suicidal ideation, given that she is at increased risk for suicide.

It is important to remember that this social work intervention process is about helping Lydia to become comfortable with her sexual identity, whether it turns out that she identifies as heterosexual or lesbian. It is not the social worker's job to judge Lydia or pressure her to try and alter her sexual orientation. The social worker may be the first person she talks to about her situation and, as such, the social worker is vital in helping Lydia to normalize her situation so that she will eventually feel comfortable coming out.

Case study #3

Witnessing or Experiencing Wartime Trauma

BY JAMIE MORTENSEN AND SUSAN KERN FROM THE US

After losing their home amidst warfare in Somalia, Fatima (14 years old) and her family were forced to flee to a refugee camp in Kenya. During their journey, Fatima's mother was raped and killed in an attack by two soldiers. Two days later, her father was killed in a crossfire shooting. Those events left Fatima as the sole caretaker of her three younger siblings.

In the Kenyan refugee camp, Fatima was faced with the hardships of taking on her new role as parent and protector to her younger siblings, while she too had become an orphan. At the same time, Fatima continued to live in constant fear regarding where she would find food for them all, and how she would be able to prevent her siblings from being harmed since the violence and troubles continued around them. Almost all of Fatima's extended family had either been lost in transit from Somalia to Kenya, or had already migrated to the US prior to their arrival—all except for one aunt, who had been caught and held hostage by soldiers for two years until she reached their camp in Kenya.

After six years in camp, and learning how to manage the process of daily living and, essentially, surviving as an older sister of three in hostile circumstances, Fatima, now 20 years old, was notified by workers from the United Nations that she and two of her siblings would be included in the next cohort of people to migrate to the US. She was told there was no room this time for her youngest brother, now seven years old, so he would stay behind with her aunt until the next cohort, which he would join to come and meet her in the US.

Now in the US for three months, Fatima has not heard anything about her youngest brother. She is having a difficult time learning the logistics about living in this new country, especially as a guardian, and is extremely worried about what might have happened with her brother. She has no way of making money and is only now considering how sad she is about everything that happened in Somalia and Kenya. She has heard about how Americans think all refugees must have problems with post-traumatic stress, so she refuses to talk to anyone about it since they might think she has more problems than she really does. She has a refugee resettlement case worker, a social worker, who asks her what is wrong.

Witnessing or Experiencing Wartime Trauma: A Social Worker from the US Responds

BY NATALIE LECY

Prevalence and Incidence

In 2010, estimates by the United Nations High Commissioner for Refugees (UNHCR) indicated that there were 15.4 million refugees in the world. Most of these refugees are hosted by developing countries. However, of the world's advanced economies, the US has the largest formal resettlement program (Center for Applied Linguistics, 2006). Consequently, of all the members of the Organization for Economic Cooperation and Development (OECD), which includes most of the world's advanced economies and emerging economies such as Japan, Canada, Germany, China, India, and Australia, the US has hosted more refugees than any of the others (Kerwin, 2011; US Department of State, n.d). The Office of Refugee Resettlement (ORR) (n.d) indicates that between 5 and 35 per cent of refugees in the US have experienced torture of some sort.

Research abounds showing that, among refugee populations, people with experiences of trauma owing to war and conflict are common (Begic

& McDonald, 2006; Ellis, MacDonald, Lincoln & Cabral, 2008). Fazel, Wheeler and Danesh (2005) conducted a meta-analysis of 20 studies involving 7,000 refugees, 4,668 of whom were residents in the US. Data from their analysis indicated that, of the present refugees residing in the US, about 50,000 out of 500,000 had post-traumatic stress disorder.

Country Policies

The US was one of the first countries to sign and ratify the United Nations' 1951 Refugee Convention. Over the course of time, there have been many policies regulating which and how many refugees are allowed into the country. This number and from which country varies annually (Haines, 2010; The University of Utah Honors Think Tank on Immigration, 2007). The most current figure for 2011 is 80,000 (Kerwin, 2011; US Department of State, n.d).

Notable among the country's policies is the Refugee Act of 1980, signed into law by President Carter on 17 March 1980. The purpose of the Act was to make institutional provisions for the resettlement of refugees. It was instrumental in the establishment of the Federal Refugee Resettlement Program. The program was established with the intent of building the capacity of refugees for independence and economic self-sufficiency within the shortest possible time on arrival in the US (Kennedy, 1981; The Refugee Act 1980). However, the Torture Victims Relief Act of 1998 is one policy that seeks to directly address the problems of people such as refugees and asylum seekers with experience of torture. In 2001 alone, a US $7.5 million provision was made available for funding torture treatment centers (Office for Refugee Resettlement, n.d).

A Social Worker Responds

In the US, social workers are trained to address the most basic needs an individual is experiencing before focusing on more advanced needs. This method was developed by Abraham Maslow and is called "Maslow's hierarchy of needs" (Maslow, 1943). In Maslow's model, the most basic needs are considered to be *physiological* (food, water, sleep), then *safety* (security, employment, health), then *love/belonging*, then *esteem*, and finally, *self-actualization*. Thus if an individual is unable to have his/her most basic physiological needs met, there will be more energy and effort invested to address these needs before he/she can invest in other needs such as safety or human connection (Maslow, 1943).

Maslow's hierarchy of needs is pertinent for Fatima's situation because she is facing multiple obstacles spanning emotional, physical, and economic barriers. Fatima is skeptical about talking to an American about the sadness she is experiencing resulting from her experiences with the war in Somalia as well as the hardships she encountered in the refugee camps in Kenya. Due to Fatima's hesitance in talking to Americans, and because she is facing some more pressing obstacles according to Maslow's hierarchy of needs, the best path for the social worker is to start working on finding resources to meet her more basic needs.

It is beneficial in two ways to focus on these needs. First, Fatima is in need of specific resources to give her the necessary skills to succeed in the US. Second, assisting Fatima with her immediate resources will help her to establish a trusting relationship with her social worker. The best course of action for the social worker is to assess what Fatima feels to be her most urgent needs and begin there (that is to meet the client where the client is). Depending on Fatima's English skills, communication between her and her social worker might need to take place through a translator.

The case scenario states that Fatima is worried about her youngest brother who remained in the Kenyan refugee camp. The social worker could assist Fatima with contacting her aunt and youngest brother. Hopefully, the aunt would have some information from the United Nations on when they are supposed to migrate to the US. If the aunt does not have this information, the social worker should contact other appropriate organizations (such as the United Nations and lawyers/legal professionals in refugee resettlement agencies) that may have information on when Fatima's relatives are scheduled to leave the Kenyan refugee camp for the US. It is important for the social worker to make sure that the youngest brother and aunt are still scheduled to come to the US. If they are already scheduled to come, the social worker should find out when and where they are arriving, as well as verifying that the aunt and brother are scheduled to arrive in the same city as Fatima so that they can be reunited.

The process of tracking the locations of the aunt and brother as well as determining their schedule for arriving in the US could be done with Fatima's participation. If Fatima is not part of the process, then the information should be relayed to her as soon as it becomes available to the social worker. If Fatima is involved in the process of ensuring her relatives' arrival in the US, the experience could help Fatima establish more trust in the social worker because they would be actively working together. Further, collaborating with Fatima could help to empower her in addition to building her capacity to navigate the US systems.

Another concern Fatima expressed in the case scenario was the responsibility of being a parent in a new country. The social worker could explore how Fatima feels about her role as a parent and if she needs any support in that role. The social worker could ask Fatima what the school systems and education were like in Somalia, and in the refugee camp in Kenya, and explore what similarities and differences in education Fatima has experienced in the US. It would be important for the social worker to determine what Fatima's understanding of the US school system is and assess if she has any questions related to it. Orientation about the rights of parents and children in the US would be helpful because they are different from other countries and it would be necessary to address any misconceptions. The social worker should assess how Fatima's siblings in the US are adjusting, as well as ensure that the younger children are enrolled in school and have the necessary resources to participate in the education system, such as uniforms, schoolbooks, school supplies, and access to transportation.

In the US, government-sponsored programs for newly-arrived refugees are available. Some of the services offered are rental assistance, food vouchers, and health insurance. As a social worker, it would be important to ensure that Fatima and her family members are enrolled in all the programs available to them, and that they learn how they work. Though these resources are available, they often come with complex policies that clients must understand and navigate to maintain benefits.

If Fatima is not fluent in English, she could benefit from an English Learning Skills class. English skills can be advantageous for a person who is seeking employment because it can be difficult in the US to find work if one does not speak English. English skills are beneficial because the individual can feel empowered and more connected to his/her community if he/she speaks the official language. Since Fatima is the guardian for her siblings, English skills could help her connect with her siblings' teachers and further help her understand the expectations the school has for them and for Fatima as their guardian.

It would be appropriate for the social worker to determine what Fatima's goals are for work and school. If Fatima is interested in school and does not have the equivalent of a high school diploma, she may want to enroll in a General Education Development (GED) program, which would help her to attain a high school diploma. This diploma could help her to secure a job because many work settings require such a qualification. In addition, a high school diploma would help Fatima enter college or university, if that is among her goals. If Fatima is interested in pursuing a high school diploma, the social worker would then have to find out which GED programs are accessible for her in regard to her location and the price she can afford. Most of the GED programs are free, but the social worker should always double-check this to make sure that Fatima is not enrolling on a program that she cannot afford.

The social worker should assess the type of employment of interest to Fatima and which jobs would best match her skills set. The worker could help Fatima create a resume highlighting her skills and past work experiences. An important topic to discuss with Fatima would be what the typical job application entails; emphasizing what would be expected of her in a job interview and in the job itself. The social worker could refer Fatima to an employment specialist in a refugee resettlement agency who would help Fatima search for job openings in the appropriate fields.

A big factor in this case scenario is Fatima's lack of extended family support. It would be important for a social worker to assess where her extended family has been relocated in the US. A social worker should assess whether Fatima has contact with any of her relatives. If she has contact with her extended family, the social worker should explore where the extended family lives, and the level of contact Fatima maintains with them. The social worker should assess if Fatima has any desire to relocate to be closer to her extended family.

There are many dimensions to consider with an individual who has newly arrived in the US. A social worker may be tempted to address Fatima's emotional distress, but if she is not ready to discuss her feelings, then the social worker will not accomplish anything. In the US, a social worker should always address the needs that the client believes are the most important. In the future, after the social worker has assisted Fatima with attaining her primary goals, Fatima may want to share her feelings of stress or sadness. At this point, the relationship will already be established and hopefully Fatima would feel safe enough to share her thoughts and feelings with her social worker. In the US, a Master's level social worker certified in the field is qualified to conduct therapy. If Fatima reaches the point where she feels comfortable to consult the social worker about her trauma experiences, the worker would be trained and qualified to address the subject.

Witnessing or Experiencing Wartime Trauma: A Social Worker from New Zealand Responds

BY LYNNE BRIGGS

Prevalence and Incidence

New Zealand society is becoming increasingly diverse to the extent that refugees and migrants from a variety of cultural backgrounds now comprise a distinct, significant, and often visible component of the demographic profile. While this has positive impacts, such as filling gaps in the labour market, there are also potential challenges, such as impact on economic and social well-being if some groups do not fare as well as others (Ministry of Social Development, 2008).

The employment rates for prime working-age migrants born in other countries are significantly lower than for the New Zealand-born population (Census New Zealand, 2006). A comparison of all sectors of society (New Zealand Immigration Service, 2004: 232, 235) found that refugees tend to have poor employment outcomes. Thus between 12 per cent and 53 per cent of refugees were employed; however, many were only working part-time with the majority of their income coming from a government benefit. As Pernice et al., (2009) point out, this in turn can lead to depression, poor mental health, and inadequate adjustment.

Country Policies

As a signatory to the United Nations' 1951 Refugee Convention and the 1967 Protocol, New Zealand meets its humanitarian obligations by providing third country resettlement to refugees, migrants and their families mandated by the United Nations High Commission (UNHCR, 1996). Estimating the exact number of refugees entering New Zealand is difficult since some come in under the "Refugee Quota system," others under family support policies, and some seek asylum. Taking all categories into account, approximately 1,250 people are offered resettlement annually (New Zealand Immigration Service, 2004).

Despite its small size, proportionally New Zealand is one of the highest migrant receiving countries in the world. Furthermore, while still relatively small in comparison to the total number of newcomers, an increasing number of people are now migrating from North East and Central Asia and Africa, all of whom, to a greater or lesser extent, tend to have the same social and mental health issues as the general population.

Under Section 22 of the New Zealand Public Health and Disability Act (2000), District Health Boards (DHBs) have a responsibility to improve, promote, and protect the health of the population within their district. Addressing the health needs of people from refugee and migrant backgrounds is an important component of meeting this responsibility. In its outline of responsibilities for the health and disability sector workforce in New Zealand, the National Mental Health Sector Standard (New Zealand Standards, 2001) also includes recommendations for working with refugees, migrants, and other ethnic clients. The laws and standards mean that while regional differences do exist in the way in which services are offered around the country, generally in the New Zealand context, refugees with psychological distress are seen in the DHB's main stream mental health services (Te Pou, 2008:9).

A Social Worker Responds

New Zealand social workers are employed in a range of practice settings and carry out a variety of functions and roles, which include case management in the DHB's mental health services. As Briggs and Cromie (2009: 225) explain, while service provision is influenced by the principles of recovery, the strengths perspective and the concept of empowerment, social work in mental health has a clinical focus. As such, social workers have a responsibility to undertake psychiatric assessments with clients, make a provisional diagnosis using the Diagnostic and Statistical Manual of Mental Disorders DSM-IV (American Psychiatric Association, 1994), and facilitate the most appropriate course of intervention. In doing so social workers also need to take into account the social context and social consequences of mental health and look beyond the symptoms and diagnosis in order to understand the impact of social, psychological, and cultural factors.

In terms of the case study, Fatima would be referred to the Refugee Mental Health Service. Once accepted into the service and allocated to a case manager, the process could involve all or some of the following:

- A comprehensive mental health assessment;
- Psychiatric consultation with a psychiatrist;
- Pharmacology intervention and medication reviews;
- Ongoing treatment using a range of intervention methods;
- A course of physiotherapy;

- A consultation with the dietician;
- Coordination advocacy with other services (e.g., Work and Income New Zealand, Work Programmes, lawyers, local Ministers of Parliament, Child, Youth and Family Services, schools, New Zealand Immigration Services, and many others entities).

When offered an assessment at the local Refugee Mental Health Service, Fatima would be advised that she can bring a support person and/or family member to attend the assessment with her. Before the assessment occurs, an appropriately trained interpreter (acceptable to Fatima) would be engaged by the mental health service. This process is essential for both the assessment and any ongoing intervention when neither the social worker nor the client speak the same language fluently. In situations where an appropriate inter-preter is unavailable in the region, then (as with any health professional in main stream health services) the social worker would have access to New Zealand Telephone Interpreter Services. This service ensures that untrained interpreters or family members would only be used to translate for a client in an emergency.

From a clinical point of view, understanding the client's perception of his/her problems is important as people from different cultures express their symptoms differently. Prior to beginning the actual assessment process, the reason for attending the service and possible outcomes would be fully explained to Fatima.

The interview questions need to be open-ended, stated clearly, and should focus on facilitation and clarification to ensure that Fatima's view of the situation is accurately captured. As the aim of the assessment is to gather information about Fatima's current functioning, any statements that require considerable interpretation need to be restated so that Fatima perfectly understands the questions. The assessment is undertaken to determine whether:

- Fatima has a mental health disorder?
- If so, what is the provisional diagnosis?
- Is she safe both emotionally and physically?
- Does Fatima require further ongoing intervention?
- If so, what is the most suitable intervention for her?
- Can this intervention be provided by the social worker?
- If not, who else should be involved in Fatima's care?
- Are there any concurrent social or health problems that need urgent attention before mental health intervention commences (e.g., physical health issues, lack of housing, finances, or social support)?
- What is the expected outcome of any intervention?

The social worker conducting the assessment obtains other collateral information (e.g., information from other medical reports), and thus the outcome is not totally reliant on Fatima's responses.

While undertaking the assessment with Fatima, the social worker is also aware from the referral letter of the traumatic events that she experienced in her country of origin, during the flight into refuge, and during her stay in the refugee camp. Additionally, while having to adapt and adjust to a new cultural environment herself, Fatima has also become the sole parent and financial provider for her younger siblings. The issue is further complicated by the worry that she is experiencing about her younger brother.

As Smith (2003: 72) highlights, refugees may have issues of trust with government and authority figures, including heath professionals. That seems to be the case for Fatima as, to date, she has refused to talk about her problems since she is fearful she may be seen as having more problems than she really does. This fear makes building an effective relationship all the more crucial.

Once the assessment has been completed, any intervention planning would be done in conjunction with Fatima and, where appropriate, her family. The planning would depend on the outcome of the psychiatric assessment and intervention may involve all, or any, of the options discussed above. Certainly coordination and advocacy with other services would form a major part of the intervention plan. This step is where case management is particularly important since refugees often find it difficult to access services on their own behalf.

In Fatima's case, it appears that she needs assistance in securing financial support for her family. This access could be achieved by the social worker contacting the Work and Income Services New Zealand (WINZ), which provides benefits to people in need, to ensure that Fatima receives her full benefit entitlement.

Furthermore, the social worker may approach the New Zealand Immigration Service (NZIMS) to determine whether Fatima's younger brother is indeed included in the next cohort coming to the country. The provision of a psychiatric report explaining the negative impact the situation is having on her mental health may assist NZIMS in their decision making process.

As well as needing to build an effective relationship with Fatima, the social worker needs to recognize symptoms of potential mental health disorders as outlined in the DSM-IV (American Psychiatric Association, 1994). In doing so, the biological, social, psychological, and cultural factors that may be affecting Fatima's mental health would be taken into account. The social worker would then work with Fatima to identify appropriate intervention goals. These steps would include liaising and advocating with other services to ensure that the client is kept fully informed about the situation of her younger brother, has access to appropriate resources, and receives full access to benefits available to her.

Exercises

Discussion Questions

1   How can social workers affirm individuals' human rights while working within legal and cultural systems which judge clients' sexual orientation as wrong? What approaches should social workers take in this case?
2   What strategies should social workers use when working with multiple professionals on a case to ensure timely and effective dispensation of client care?
3   What are "best practices" for working with juvenile delinquents? How might this differ by country or culture?
4   Consider the role of law enforcement agencies and non-governmental entities working with populations who have experienced trauma. Are there cultural parameters that constitute a hindrance as to how these professional groups respond to incidents of trauma? How do social workers and law enforcement agents work together in your home country when these issues occur?

Classroom Exercises

1   In small groups, student should create a treatment plan for Hunter. If the students were the social worker in that case, what should happen? Then discuss as a whole class how these treatment plans fit within students' country and cultural contexts. Discuss how the social work intervention is a reflection of culture?
2   Students should work in small groups to discuss the following issues. How are the UN Conventions linked to social work and treating victims of trauma? Do these conventions say anything about how social workers are to engage and/or practice in this arena?

References

Adiatu, D. (2009). "Stonewall riots: The beginning of the LGBT movement." Retrieved from http://www.civilrights.org/archives/2009/06/449-stonewall.html

American Psychiatric Association. (1994). *Diagnostic and Statistical Manual of Mental Disorders, 4th Edition*. American Psychiatric Association, Washington, DC.

American Psychological Association [APA] Task Force on Appropriate Therapeutic Responses to Sexual Orientation. (2009). *Report of the Task Force on Appropriate Therapeutic Responses to Sexual Orientation*. Washington, D.C: American Psychological Association.

Andrews, D. & Bonta, J. (2010). "Rehabilitating criminal justice policy and practice." *Psychology, Public Policy, and Law*, 16, 39–55.

Attipoe, D. (2004). "West Africa project to combat HIV/AIDS and STI (WAPCAS) (First Draft): Revealing the pandora box or playing the ostrich? A situational appraisal of men having sex with men in the Accra metropolitan area and its environs – Ghana." Retrieved from www.freewebs.com/african-rapport/MSMReport3%5B1%5D.doc.

Bagley, C., & Tremblay, P. (2000). "Elevated rates of suicidal behavior in gay, lesbian and bisexual youth." *Research Trends*, 21 (3), 111–17.

Begic, S., & McDonald, T. W. (2006). "The psychological effects of exposure to wartime trauma in Bosnian residents and refugees: Implications for treatment and service provision." *International Journal of Mental Health and Addiction*, 4, 319–29.

Briggs, L. & Cromie, B. (2009). "Social Work Mental Health in New Zealand." In M. Connolly & Center for Applied Linguistics (2006). *Cultural orientation for refugees: A handbook for US trainers*. Washington, DC: Author.

Browne, C. & Mills, C. (2001). "Theoretical frameworks: Ecological model, strengths perspective, and empowerment theory." In R. Fong & S. Furuto (Eds.), *Culturally competent practice: Skills, interventions, and evaluations*. (pp. 10–32). Boston, MA: Allyn and Bacon.

Center for Applied Linguistics (2006). *Cultural orientation for refugees: A handbook for US trainers*. Washington, DC: Author.

Chesney-Lind, M., Pasko, L., Marker, N., & Fiaui, P. (2003). Youth service center evaluation research volume II: A report to the twenty-second Hawai'i state legislature. Center for Youth Research, Social Science Research Institute, University of Hawai'i at Manoa.

Davis, R. L. (2005). "Risk and protective factors for Pacific Islander youth in Utah." (Unpublished doctoral dissertation). University of Utah, Salt Lake City.

Department of Social Welfare (DSW) (2011). Department of social welfare records. Kumasi: DSW.

Ellis, B., MacDonald, H. Z., Lincoln, A. K., & Cabral, H. J. (2008). "Mental health of Somali adolescent refugees: The role of trauma, stress, and perceived discrimination." *Journal Of Consulting And Clinical Psychology*, 76, 184–93.

Fazel, M., Wheeler, J., & Danesh, J. (2005). "Prevalence of serious mental disorder in 7000 refugees resettled in western countries: A systematic review." *The Lancet*, 365 (9467), 1309–14.

Frankfort-Nachmias, C., & Leon-Guerrero, A. (1997). *Social statistics for a diverse society*. Thousand Oaks, CA:Pine Forge Press.

Ghana (n.d). Retrieved from <http://paei.state.gov/documents/organization/160124.pdf>

Haines, D. W. (2010). *Safe haven: A history of refugees in America*. Sterling, VA: Kumarian.

Janes, C. R. (1990). *Migration, social change, and health: A Samoan community in urban California*. Stanford, CA: Stanford University Press.

Joe, K. & Chesney-Lind, M. (1995). "'Just Every Mother's Angel': An analysis of gender and ethnic variations in youth gang membership." *Gender & Society*, 9, 408–31.

Kennedy, E. M. (1981). "Refugee Act of 1980." *International Migration Review*, 15, 141–56.

Kerwin, D. (2011). *The faltering US refugee. Protection system: Legal and policy responses to refugees, asylum seekers, and others in need of protection*. Washington, DC: Migration Policy Institute.

Lee, E. (2002). *Cultural diversity series: Meeting the mental health needs of Asian and Pacific Islander Americans*. Alexandria, VA: National Technical Assistance Center for State Mental Health Planning.

Lord Beveridge Report. (1944). In S. Opoku, (1991). "Volunteerism, Colonialism and Social Work in Ghana." (Unpublished Thesis)

Luckie, M. S. (n.d). "Somewhere over the rainbow." Retrieved from http://journalism.berkeley.edu/projects/mm/luckie/rainbow.html

Martinson, R. (1974). "What works? Questions and answers about prison reform." *The Public Interest*, 35, 22–54.

Maslow, A. H. (1943). "A theory of human motivation." *Psychological Review*, 50 (4), 370–96.

Ministry of Social Development, New Zealand (2010). *Social Report*. Retrieved from http://www.socialreport.msd.govt.nz/

Mokuau, N. (1991). *Handbook of social services for Asian and Pacific Islanders*, Westport, CT: Greenwood Press.

Morgan, K. S., & Nerison, R. M. (1993). "Homosexuality and psychopolitics: An historical overview." *Psychotherapy*, 30 (1), 133–40.

Nelson, J. A. (1994). "Comment on special issue on adolescence." *American Psychologist*, 49 (6), 523–24.

Nelson, T. S., & Thomas, F. N. (Eds.) (2009). *Handbook of solution-focused brief therapy*. Binghamton, NY: Hawthorne.

New Zealand Immigration Service (2004). *Refugee Voices: A Journey Towards Resettlement*. Department of Labour.

Office of Refugee Resettlement (ORR) (n.d). "Services for survivors of torture." Retrieved from http://www.acf.hhs.gov/programs/orr/programs/services_survivors_torture.htm

Opoku, S. (1991). Volunteerism, colonialism and social work in Ghana. (Unpublished Thesis).

Pernice R., Trlin A., Henderson A., North, N. & Skinner, M. (2009). "Employment Status, Duration of Residence and Mental Health Among Skilled Migrants To New Zealand: Results of a Longitudinal Study." *International Journal of Social Psychiatry*, 55 (3): 272–87

Puzzanchera, C. (2009). "Juvenile arrests 2008." *OJJDP Juvenile Justice Bulletin (December 2009)*. Retrieved from https://www.ncjrs.gov/pdffiles1/ojjdp/228479.pdf

Savin-Williams, R. C., (1994). "Verbal and physical abuse as stressors in the lives of lesbian, gay male, and bisexual youths: Associations with school problems, running away, substance abuse, prostitution and suicide." *Journal of Consulting and Clinical Psychology*, 62 (2), 261–69.

Smith, Michelle (2003). *Health care for refugees, View Point*. NSW Refugee Health Service, Australia.

Te Pou. (2008). "Refugee and Migrant Mental Health and Addiction Research Agenda for New Zealand 2008–2012." *Te Pou: The National Centre of Mental Health Research, Information and Workforce Development*. Auckland, New Zealand.

The University of Utah Honors Think Thank on Immigration (2007). "Immigration in context: A resource guide for Utah." Retrieved from http://www.econ.utah.edu/~jameson/assets/Resource%20Guide.pdf

Thoreson, R., & Cook, S. (Eds.) (2011). *Nowhere to turn: Blackmail and extortion of LGBT people in Sub-Saharan Africa*. Brooklyn, NY: IGLHRC.

US Department of State (n.d.). The US refugee admissions program. Retrieved from http://www.state.gov/g/prm/c26471.htm

Umbreit, M. S., & Armour, M. P. (2010). *Restorative justice dialogues: An essential guide for research and practice*. New York: Springer.

UNHCR (2011). "World refugee day: UNHCR report finds 80 per cent of world's refugees in developing countries." Retrieved from http://www.unhcr.org/4dfb66ef9.html

UNHCR (1996). "Convention and 1967 Protocols Relating to the Status of Refugees. Public Information Section." United Nations High Commission for Refugees. Retrieved from http://untreaty.un.org/cod/avl/ha/prsr/prsr.html

United Nations International Children's Emergency Fund (2011). Protect and support affected children: The challenge. Retrieved from http://www.childinfo.org/hiv_aids_children_affected.html

Vakalahi, H. F. O. (2009). "Pacific Islander American students: Caught between a rock and a hard place?" *Children and Youth Services Review*, 31, 1258–63.

Wasserman G. A., Keenan, K., Tremblay, R. E., Coie, J. D., Herrenkohl, T. I., Loeber, R., et al. (2003). "Risk and protective factors of child delinquency." Child Delinquency Bulletin Series: Office of Juvenile Justice and Delinquency Prevention. Retrieved from http://www.ghana.gov.gh/living/constitution/chapter05.php

9 | Substance Abuse

By Gloria Jacques

Substance use and abuse is prevalent across cultures. It is a problem not limited to any particular society, gender, age structure, or socio-economic class. The use of drugs and substances such as alcohol, cannabis, and opium are ancient practices engendered by sociocultural factors in many societies (Asuni & Pela, 1986; WHO, 2005; Willis, 2006). Consumption and use of alcoholic beverages and drugs can be a contributory factor to family violence, causing family members to often live in fear and suffer, as do the abusers, from mental disorders (Fals-Stewart, Birchler, & O'Farrell, 1999). Substance abuse by parents is a risk factor for similar abuse by their children (WHO, 2004). In developed countries, parental abuse of substances may at times be a reason for the placement of children in foster care (Dore, Doris & Wright, 1995) since it undermines caregiver capacity to provide optimal care to children, which may lead to delinquency and "street-ism" in children (Baron, 1999). In addition, treatment modalities for cases of drug and substance abuse may vary depending on locality. In some societies, the hope for treatment is minimal because adequately trained professionals to deal with these issues are lacking. In other nations, individuals have the benefit of assistance by professionals and skilled therapists. The issues around substance abuse and treatment modalities are explored in the cases and analyses in this chapter.

Case study #1

Getting Someone to Acknowledge that He/She Has a Problem with Substance Abuse

BY ANITA NEAL & TARA TULLEY FROM THE US

Cathy is a 23-year-old, unmarried female who is ordered by a judge to begin weekly outpatient substance treatment. She comes to see a social worker with Linda, her sister, who has temporary custody of Cathy's four children (ages ranging from three to nine years). Linda is frustrated because Cathy is an alcoholic who frequently puts her children in dangerous living situations, and leaves open bottles of alcohol in the home accessible to the children. Linda says that Cathy leaves the children alone for days at a time with the nine-year-old caring for the younger children. Linda says the nine-year-old boy's teachers are concerned because he is frequently absent from school. Cathy has a boyfriend who comes and goes from the home. He physically and verbally abuses Cathy, and Linda suspects he has sexually abused the three-year-old based on some inappropriate sexual behaviors she shows in the home.

Linda has cared for Cathy's children before when Cathy has disappeared for long periods of time, and then reappeared and wanted her children back. Linda wants Cathy to recognize the problems her drug use are causing and either commit to treatment or give Linda permanent guardianship of the children.

Cathy is pregnant with her fifth child, and Linda is concerned that Cathy is still drinking and having unprotected sex with multiple partners. Cathy does not think there is a problem because she receives state support with housing and food. She does not want to give up custody and lose the assistance.

Linda has supported Cathy financially and taken her children for periods of time to help Cathy get back on her feet. Cathy sometimes told Linda she was leaving her children with her to obtain residential treatment when she was really spending time with sexual partners, using alcohol, and having parties. Linda says that Cathy needs help to give up her children so that Linda can care for them on a permanent basis.

Getting Someone to Acknowledge that He/She Has a Problem with Substance Abuse: A Social Worker from Brazil Responds

BY ROBERTA UCHOA

Prevalence and Incidence

The pattern of drinking score related to alcohol-attributable burden of disease is considered medium in Brazil, with alcohol-attributable deaths as a percentage of total deaths ranging from 5–10 per cent (especially cirrhosis of the liver and road traffic accidents) (World Health Organization [WHO], 2011). Within the population, 75 per cent have used alcohol once, 50 per cent have been drunk in the last year, 38 per cent have been drunk in the last month, and 12 per cent are alcohol dependent (Senad, 2005). Males drink more in all categories than females and people with less education have a 2.1 times greater relative risk of alcohol dependence than those with higher education. Female alcohol dependence is around 7 per cent. However, between 2006 and 2009, more females than males reported at least one episode of excessive drinking in the past 30 days. Prevalence of heavy episodic drinking (15 to 85+ years) is 32 per cent for males and 10 per cent for females. Brazilian drinkers enjoy drinking beer (54 per cent), spirits (40 per cent), wine (5 per cent), and other beverages (1 per cent) (Andrade, Walters, Gentil, & Laurenti, 2002). Although the national legal minimum age for on- and off-premises sales of alcoholic drinks is 18 years, exposure to alcohol begins early and binge drinking among young people is a major public health issue (Schmidt et al., 2011). Treatment for alcohol addiction is not compulsory in the public health sector unless there is a criminal offence involved in an alcohol abuse or dependence case. According to Brazilian drug law, only illegal drug users could be afforded compulsory treatment at an outpatient facility or given penalties such as compulsory community work or the payment of a fine (Drug Law, 2006).

There are no reliable data in Brazil related to loss or suspension of parental custody and guidance because of alcohol addiction. However, in recent years, because of the increase in the number of crack cocaine users in the country, more and more cases of loss or suspension of parental custody and guidance are being identified by drug addiction services, suggesting that research in this field should be developed.

Country Policies

In 1988, after 24 years of military dictatorship, the Brazilian Congress passed a new Federal Constitution defining, among other things, many social rights as well as duties of the federal, state, and municipal public sectors to individuals. Social security (including health, social welfare, and social retirement protection), education, culture, sport and leisure, science and technology, family, children, young people, and the elderly all received a new set of definitions and regulations to provide for well-being and social justice in Brazil. At this time (1988), a national debate is being held on the subject of mental ill health, which stimulated the development of new regulations for the mental health sector, deinstitutionalization processes, innovative community care practices, and clear definitions of mental illness. The health, drug addiction, social welfare, and child and adolescent protection systems were all developed based on these approaches (Brazilian Federal Constitution, 1988).

Health Organic Law (known as Sanitary Reform) defined health as a state resulting from access to essential social needs, goods, and services, and declared that the provision of health should be delivered through a Unified Health System (SUS). New drug addiction regulations were introduced between 2000 and the present incorporating a more tolerant approach to illegal drugs such as cessation of incarceration for drug users, harm reduction strategies, and drop-in, community, and housing protection services (Health Organic Law, 1990a; Psychiatric Reform Law, 2001; Ministry of Health, 2003).

The Child and Adolescent Treaty (ECA) determines that young people have fundamental rights to physical, mental, moral, spiritual, and social development in free and dignifying conditions. According to the ECA, "every child or adolescent has the right to be raised and educated in the midst of his family and, exceptionally, in a foster family, in such a way as to ensure family and community life in an environment free of the presence of persons dependent on narcotic substances." In suspected cases of mistreatment threatening or violating child and adolescent rights, notification is compulsory to a local Tutelary Council (Conselho Tutelar). The obligations of this Council include public care services for minors, parental counseling, and referring proven cases of disrespect of child and adolescent rights to the judicial system (Child and Adolescent Treaty, 1990b).

Brazil has currently nearly 80,000 social workers, mostly working with the formulation, planning, execution, and/or research of public policies including mental health and drug addiction. Most health, drug addiction, social welfare, and child and adolescent public protection services in Brazil have social workers as part of their multi-disciplinary teams. However, despite meaningful progress in the social protection framework, social policies relating to public health, social welfare, and child and adolescent protection are weak, as is the family's ability to provide care to relatives in need, with a special burden for women who are most commonly the caregivers.

A Social Worker Responds

Brazilian social workers are oriented to follow national social policy guidelines as well as their professional ethical code of conduct. At an outpatient Psychosocial Care Centre (CAP) for alcohol and drug abuse, Cathy would be interviewed by a social worker using motivational interviewing techniques to learn about her life history, especially her drinking problem and previous treatment, and try to help her to engage in further therapy. The social worker would explain to Cathy the availability of public treatment options (part- or full-time day care, 30 days inpatient care at a therapeutic shelter, and intensive care in a general hospital for detoxification). She would refer Cathy for a prenatal examination at the nearest maternal care unit, recommending her to have HIV and other sexually transmitted disease tests. Cathy would be asked about her children's social living conditions in relation to nourishment, housing standards, school attendance, exposure to alcohol and other drug use, physical and mental abuse, and any kind of violence.

The social worker would inform Cathy that a home visit would be necessary so that he/she could hear from the children what their needs were. She would also remind Cathy of all stipulated requirements in caring for her children, especially those stated in the (ECA), and the possibility of state financial support. Although alcohol addiction treatment is not compulsory in the country, Cathy is under a legal order and has to decide if she will accept therapy. If she does not do so, Cathy would be referred back to the legal system and the social worker would have to report to the Tutelary Council nearest Cathy's place of residence about the living conditions of her children. In response to the legal order the social worker, along with health professionals at the CAP, and regarding gender issues, he/she would create an Individual Therapeutic Project with Cathy stating her rights and obligations during her treatment at the health facility.

During Cathy's treatment, the social worker would make home visits to identify improvement or otherwise in the social development of the children. A social worker in Brazil would make every effort to keep the family together through information and referrals to the available Brazilian social protection systems, especially for the underprivileged and those with drug dependency.

Temporary or permanent loss of the children during treatment could militate against Cathy's progress. During treatment, if threats or violations of the children's rights were suspected or proven, the social worker would report the case to the Tutelary Council, which would take responsibility for the care of the children and, if necessary, institute legal procedures to give permanent guardianship of Cathy's children to her sister, Linda.

Getting Someone to Acknowledge That He/She Has a Problem with Substance Abuse: A Social Worker from Botswana Responds

BY MAITHAMAKO MOLOJWANE

Prevalence and Incidence

There are no available statistics on alcohol and drug abuse in Botswana, but there is related evidence that substantial problems exist. In response to this perceived issue, the government has recently introduced an alcohol levy to support programs assisting those who are affected by the 'by-products' of substance use and abuse. Legislation has been passed to limit the opening hours of bars and other places serving alcohol, and "shebeen queens" (women who sell liquor from their homes) are no longer allowed to do so. There are Alcoholics Anonymous (AA) groups in the only two cities in Botswana—Gaborone (the capital) and Francistown (in the north of the country). Police roadblocks are currently operating along major roads and breathalyzer tests are being conducted on a regular basis. Furthermore, fines for driving while under the influence of alcohol or drugs have recently been increased in an attempt to deter those who do so (thereby putting their own lives, and the lives of others, at risk).

Country Policies

Botswana is a former British Protectorate which gained independence in 1966. Most of its policies were inherited from Britain and thus not totally relevant to the state of Botswana today. For instance, the Adoption of Children Act (28:01) of 1952 is still in force although it is in the process of amendment (2012). Children are mainly cared for under the traditional kinship system which, although considerably weakened, is still being used for children in need of care, especially in rural areas. Many grandparents are taking care of their orphaned and other vulnerable grandchildren. Upon the death of grandparents, the existing aunts and uncles are the first people to be consulted or contacted to assess their willingness to take in children who are in need of care and protection. However, the AIDS pandemic and other diseases have considerably weakened this support system. If there are no relatives alive or willing to care for the children, other alternatives such as institutional care, although limited in the country, can be sought. A statutory foster care program, planned for over a period of 13 years, is only now (2012) nearing implementation.

In Botswana, caregiving by family is widely preferred to institutional care. In the cultural context, people of Cathy's age often migrate to cities and towns, leaving behind their young children under the care of elderly relatives. The relatives, grandmothers in particular, in turn expect to be rewarded for this service, but in reality most if not all of the young mothers who migrate to urban centers do not send money to assist in caring for their children back home. The Ministry of Local Government, through its Department of Social Services, provides some measure of social welfare services to the children including clothing, school uniforms, and food.

Social work's current status in Botswana is characterized by professionals from different cadres such as adult education, home economics, and community development, as well as those who have qualified as social workers. The profession is currently faced with the challenge of work overload leading to lack of sufficient time to meet all the clients' needs. As a result, most are reduced to dealing largely with presenting issues, at the expense of a critical analysis of the root causes of problems, leading to the development of a dependency syndrome on the part of service users, especially destitute persons.

Every village, town, and city has the services of a social worker, employed by the local authority while fewer are employed by NGOs. At local authority level, a lone social worker in a village or rural area is expected to perform a wide array of duties. Specialization in government service is rare, although it is much more common in non-governmental organizations. In addition to the problem of wide areas of coverage, a government social work practitioner in the field is faced with a lack of reasonable office accommodation and transport.

A Social Worker Responds

A social worker in Botswana would consider Cathy's children to be in need of care and protection under the Children's Act of 2009. The social worker would mainly apply Section 42 of this Act, which defines a child in need of protection as one who has no parent, other relative, or guardian, or who has such people in their lives but they are unable to care for the child or exercise proper control due to mental or physical incapacitation. The Act further states that a child in need of protection is a child who is living under circumstances that are likely to adversely affect his/her emotional and psychosocial well-being.

Reporting of a case of children in need of protection is dealt with under Section 43 of the Children's Act, which states that any person believing that a child is in need of protection should immediately make a report to a social worker or police officer in the district in which the child is resident. The official would then investigate the allegation and, if they are satisfied that the child is in need of protection, a social worker would compile a report containing recommendations on future action to be submitted to the Children's Court, which is a magistrate's court specifically constituted for that purpose. If he/she believes that the child is likely to suffer harm if not removed to a place of safety, the social worker will immediately do so.

With regard to the present case, the social worker would first find out if Linda is fit to care for Cathy's children. This determination can be established through the use of psychometric tests such as the clinical anger scale or the presenting self-esteem scale. Then the social worker can address the frustration that Linda is experiencing. In addition, the social worker would assess other family systems in the best interest of the children and possibly arrange for psychometric testing of the nine-year-old. On the basis of the results, the social worker would arrange for appropriate therapy for him (for example, play therapy) since he has endured stress as a result of being a parent or caregiver at an early developmental stage.

The social worker would also make an arrangement to meet the guidance and counseling teacher at the boys' school to ensure a continuum of care, and to find out how the child can be assisted with the time lost through absenteeism. The social worker would also examine how the other three children have been affected and construct a baseline model which would indicate resulting problems to be tackled. These may include inappropriate sexual behaviors resulting from sexual abuse; loss of attachment from having been left on their own; and learned behaviors such as drinking, smoking, and having multiple partners which may be imitated by the children.

The social worker would then design an intervention strategy and use models such as cognitive behavior therapies to treat the children. These actions would be carried out in a safe environment which has been identified by the professional. As the proposed statutory foster care program has not yet been implemented, the children might be placed in an alternative care facility (of which there are very few in Botswana, especially for short-term care), or with Linda, other suitable relatives, or neighbors. Furthermore, the social worker would refer Cathy to a health practitioner to deal with, among other things, the issue of pregnancy, alcohol abuse, and unprotected sex, especially since there is a risk of her contracting HIV which is prevalent in the country.

The social worker would carry out a family assessment in this case, and if it indicates that Cathy is not fit to look after her children, the social worker would then apply for a protection order from the Children's Court. The application would be filed with the court specifying the grounds upon which the order was made. In Cathy's case, the application would be on the grounds that the children are found to be in need of care and protection.

An assessment report would be attached to the application. In the report, the social worker would recommend that Linda be given immediate custody/legal guardianship of the children for a period of six months while Cathy's multiple problems are being assessed. The report would also recommend that Cathy be denied visitation rights to the children for the first three months to enable them to adjust to their new circumstances.

The social worker would regularly visit Linda to see how the children are coping. When the children are with Linda, the social worker would arrange for a medical examination of the three-year-old who is suspected of having being sexually abused by Cathy's boyfriend. Childline would provide counseling and play therapy which would assist the child to disclose what had happened to her.

If both the medical examination and the child's disclosure prove beyond reasonable doubt that the three-year-old has been sexually abused, the social worker would file an application before the Children's Court under Section 57 of the Children's Act of 2009 which states that any parent who induces, coerces, or encourages a child to commit a sexually immoral act shall be guilty of an offence and liable to imprisonment for between two to five years or a substantial fine.

The social worker would also apply for material support for Linda so as to reduce the financial burden of having to care for extra members of the family. Linda's economic status would be assessed and, if she needed it, help would be provided in accordance with the Revised National Policy on Destitute Persons (2002). According to the policy, Cathy's children would qualify to be assisted as vulnerable children with food, clothing, or medical and educational necessities.

The social worker would also provide counseling for Cathy and link her to other relevant agencies which would be of help in addressing her problems. These might include the Sbrana Psychiatric Hospital, which is the institution providing treatment for alcohol and substance abuse in Botswana. There are no rehabilitation centers which specifically deal with substance abuse. However, Alcoholics Anonymous (AA) does exist and could prove to be of assistance to Cathy, as might Lifeline, which assists people with a variety of complex and challenging issues.

Case study #2

Identifying Substance Abuse Issues in One's Partner

BY CAROLYN STERRETT & MEGAN O'KEEFE FROM THE US

Lisa and Steve are a middle-aged couple living in an urban environment. They are a middle class couple raising two young children. They have been moderate social drinkers for the previous eight years of their marriage. Over the past year, Lisa has begun to notice a change in Steve. He has been sleeping through his alarm in the morning, getting up very groggy, occasionally wetting the bed, and experiencing severe morning nausea, headaches, and tremors. His alcohol consumption has increased from a few beers a night to at least twelve. She has also noticed him drinking in the morning before work. When she expresses her concern, he explains his behavior by saying he just needed a "pick me up," a little help from the alcohol to get up in the morning.

Steve was formerly a very involved father. He would often play with the children, read them books, and help Lisa with daily child-rearing tasks. Recently, she has noticed Steve withdrawing from the children and becoming irritated when they seek his attention. This behavior is out of character for him. He works at a large grocery store. He is responsible for moving pallets with a forklift and occasionally interacting with customers. Over the past few months he has had a couple of accidents while driving the forklift. He was involved in a collision at the store between the forklift and the side of the building. Customers have also complained that he smelled of alcohol and was acting intoxicated. Eventually, Steve's behavior led to his being fired from his job. Lisa has also found paraphernalia for marijuana use in the garage. He has returned from the garage appearing high and smelling of marijuana. His use of an illegal drug concerns her, especially because of the children. Because of his increase in alcohol consumption, withdrawal from the family, job loss, and marijuana use, Lisa has come to the conclusion that Steve has developed a substance abuse problem. Lisa has decided to approach Steve about his problem. She asks him to go with her to see a social worker.

Identifying Substance Abuse Issues in One's Partner: A Social Worker from South Korea Responds

BY SO RAH PARK & KWON HO CHOI

Prevalence and Incidence

Alcohol abuse is a serious social problem in Korea. Adult per capita consumption of pure alcohol from 2003—2005 was 14.8 liters, placing the country in the highest consumer group in the world (World Health Organization [WHO], 2011). Heavy episodic drinking among adult males was 23.2 per cent and adult females 8.5 per cent in 2008 (Ministry of Health and Social Welfare of Korea, 2011). The rate of help seeking among people with alcohol dependency is only 4.5 per cent in Korea (Ministry of Health and Social Welfare of Korea, 2011), which is much lower than the US (Hasin, Stinson, Ogburn, & Grant, 2007).

Country Policies

As risk factors of high consumption of alcohol, lack of regulating laws, as well as the availability of alcohol in social contexts, are significant (Hawkins, Catalano, & Miller, 1992). It should be noted that Koreans are comparatively permissive towards heavy drinking and are likely to rely on alcohol to enhance social relationships. Also, laws relating to the purchasing of alcohol and treatment and rehabilitation of abusers are not well organized. An alcohol abuse policy, The Bluebird Plan, is in its infancy in the country, having been formulated in 2006. However, its effectiveness is in question (Yoon, 2010). The brief intervention approach before, or soon after, the onset of alcohol-related problems (Room, Babor, & Rehm, 2005) is promising, but most resources have been invested in the treatment of severe alcohol problems (Ministry of Health and Social Welfare of Korea, 2011). For these reasons, alcohol abusers do not seek professional help until they have severe physical problems, such as cirrhosis of the liver or road accident injuries.

A Social Worker Responds

Social workers often encounter clients who deny their alcohol problems. Because of lack of insight, clients do not seek professional help since they believe that they are able to escape from alcohol-related problems on their own (Schober & Annis, 1996). Despite social problems such as tardiness at the workplace or physical abuse of partners, family members have difficulty in recognizing the severity of alcohol abuse. For these reasons, patients with alcohol problems detected by related agencies are fewer than those detected through non-alcohol-related interventions in Korea (Shin, 2002).

In this case, Steve and his family may first meet medical doctors, since the mental health tradition in Korea emphasizes an interdisciplinary team approach led by a medical doctor, with few patients having access initially to social workers. Medical practitioners are leaders of teams in mental health settings and social workers participate as treatment team members at alcohol-related agencies.

The first step in the assessment process is related to identifying Steve's strengths and weaknesses and formulating goals for treatment and intervention. Motivation to change is an important factor, as are previous attempts made by the client and his family to address the situation. The worker would also consider the coping strategies and adaptation styles of Steve and his family, as well as relationships, coping mechanisms, norms, and the alcohol-related culture within the family. Life stressors and community resources and support would also be assessed. Furthermore, Steve's suicidal ideation (if any) would be explored as well as a possible history of domestic violence or child abuse in his younger years. Confidentiality is an ethical problem in some instances in Korea, especially when information is shared with team members. Once the assessment is made, care plans are drawn up by the team and these may include assistance by community mental health centers, although a majority of people with alcohol-related problems desire help from hospitals.

Steve's alcohol dependency would appear to be severe even in terms of Korea's generous alcohol acceptance culture, and thus the social worker and the mental health team may evaluate him as a high risk patient and advise hospitalization where he will receive the services of the mental health team. The first step involving withdrawal symptoms will require the emotional support and education of the client and his family by a social worker. If severe physical ailments such as hepatic cancer are present the social worker might have to assist in mobilizing resources to address financial implications which could be significant. The social worker would also administer cognitive behavioral therapy to assist Steve to cope with his craving for alcohol and adherence to an abstinence regimen. Family support is vital to ensure that the family helps Steve to adapt to his newfound lifestyle. The triangular therapeutic alliance between patient/client, family, and treatment team is a critical element in addressing alcohol dependency.

Finally, the social worker would provide follow-up services. Although Steve may be discharged from hospital, the therapeutic intervention is not terminated. A social worker may link him with self-help groups such as Alcoholics Anonymous to sustain his motivation towards abstinence. Furthermore, the worker may refer Steve to a community mental health center so that he may receive a continuum of care.

Identifying Substance Abuse Issues in One's Partner: A Social Worker from Finland Responds

BY LEENA LEINONEN, PIIA PUURUNEN, MARI SUONIO, & MARJA VÄÄNÄNEN-FOMIN

Prevalence and Incidence

Steve's case provides a challenge for a social worker since, from a Finnish point of view, he represents a new type of mixed use substance abuser (Hakkarainen & Metso, 2005). Drinking habits have traditionally been uniform and intoxication oriented, while consumers have mainly been men. Nowadays, only a small number of people are abstinent, with the majority drinking moderately and a small amount drinking excessively. Drinking patterns have changed slowly toward a European style of alcohol consumption, meaning that the popularity of strong beverages has decreased in favor of light wines, beer, and ciders. Nowadays, as in Steve and Lisa's case, people are social drinkers. The most common place to drink is at home, and couples typically drink together. However, the drinking culture is ambivalent and remains drunkenness oriented. Unlike most European countries, alcohol consumption levels have increased in recent years with the total consumption reaching 10.2 liters of pure alcohol per capita in 2009 (Mäkelä, Mustonen, & Christoffer, 2010; National Institute for Health and Welfare, 2009.)

Drug problems in Finland escalated after the mid-1990s, but since 2000 the drug markets appear to have stabilized. The dominant illegal drugs are cannabis and amphetamine. According to the most recent population study in 2008, 13 per cent of the adult population had tried cannabis at some point in their lives. Latest estimates suggest that less than one per cent of the population has a problematic case of drug use (Forsell, Virtanen, Jääskeläinen, Alho, & Partanen, 2010.) Homegrown drugs and possession of drugs for personal use are considered crimes, and account for the majority of sentences related to narcotics in Finland. The typical penalty is a fine (Kainulainen, 2009).

Country Policies

The history of legislation connected with intoxicants has focused on the control of deviant behavior and been directed at the underprivileged and poor. Intoxication has been considered a moral issue, a bad habit, an example of a lack of coping skills, and—most recently—as a social and health problem. Interventions are now justified by the individual's need for care and the perspective of human rights (Kaukonen, 2000). In Finland, the responsibility for organizing social and health services lies historically with municipalities. Seeking help for substance abuse is based on the client's own initiative to act voluntarily and under confidential conditions as compulsory treatment is seldom used (Welfare for Substance Abusers Act, 1986).

A Social Worker Responds

Responsibility for the intervention lies with Lisa as occupational health care, which normally has an important role in effective early intervention in Finland, has been lacking in Steve's case. His substance abuse problems have become so severe that they have caused physical, psychological, and social harm. Due to the severity of Steve's problems, Lisa makes an appointment for them to meet a specialized social worker at the local A-Clinic. The intoxicant clinics are generally referred to in Finland as A-Clinics and are maintained by municipalities or the A-Clinic Foundation (Paihdelinkki, 2011a).

The starting point for the social worker is to recognize Lisa and Steve's story and how they came to realize that Steve has a problem. It might take a long time for family members, and the person himself, to comprehend that something is not right. Confronting the substance abuse problem is a process that includes periods of uncertainty and doubt, worry, and fear about what is happening. The social worker can evaluate, based on the couple's story, that Steve has become a heavy user. If the situation does not change, it might lead Lisa to adopt coping strategies such as leaving home, trying to control Steve's drinking, or even participating in his use of alcohol. Yet sometimes the family can be a positive element in the recovery process (Holmila, 2001). The social worker is not just aiming to help Steve as an individual, but also recognizing and implementing a systems-oriented approach with a family-centered way of working.

Although it is clear that Steve has a problem with substance abuse, the family's story will not reveal at this point whether there are some other reasons as to why Steve has increased his alcohol intake and been smoking marijuana. Addiction problems develop differently in different people, and addiction might be a cause of many varying problems. The treatment possibilities can also be arranged to suit the individual, but the most important starting point is Steve's personal motivation (Kuusisto, 2009).

Since a social worker is proceeding with the family, he or she starts with a thorough investigation of how they are coping, and gives information about social security benefits, existing services, and possibilities for immediate detoxification. One important issue to address is whether Steve's firing was lawful and why the employer had not referred Steve to occupational health care. The social worker would advise Steve to make an appointment at the local labor force bureau.

The social worker will then recommend a period of evaluation for Steve at the A-Clinic and help him to apply for a municipality bond to cover the costs of the evaluation period. Steve's situation will be discussed by the multi-professional team at the A-Clinic, which includes a medical doctor, psychologist, social worker, and nurses. Intoxicant services in Finland are generally carried out in a multi-disciplinary and multi-professional way with the orientation of multi-disciplinary work being dialogical and equal (Seikkula & Arnkil, 2005; Mönkkönen, 2007). The theory base for the intervention varies depending on the orientation of each worker.

Psychosocial orientation is integral to all social work in Finland, which means that every social worker has the basic ability to observe and assess the overall psychological status of their clients. According to the principles of psychosocial work, every social worker is prepared to confront clients in a therapeutic manner (Granfelt, 1993; Woods & Robinson, 1996.) The most common theory bases used in Finnish intoxicant outpatient services are cognitive-behavioral, motivational, systemic, solution-focused, and neuro-linguistic programming. Others could be implemented depending on the therapist's training and the needs of the client (Päihdelinkki, 2011b).

In Steve's case, the social worker is trying to arouse his awareness of the effects of his behavior on the family. In order to do this, the social worker mainly uses motivational interviewing and the development of a dialogical relationship with Steve (Miller & Rollnick, 2002.) It is important to make Steve understand that his unpredictable behavior is confusing Lisa and their children. As the social worker and Steve continue their meetings, the themes of the interviews would cover family and social relations, housing, the financial situation, working experience and education, health issues and substance use, and daily life. Maintaining Steve's motivation and discussing further goals of the therapy is vital. During the next two to four meetings, different kinds of tools and tests will be used to increase consciousness of the problematic intoxicant use. Two commonly used tests are Alcohol Use Disorders Identification Test (AUDIT) and Short-form Alcohol Dependence Data Questionnaire (SADD). The social worker also discusses Steve's relations with his children using the Network Map tool, which is a well-known tool in social work in Finland based on the ecological systems theory of Bronfenbrenner. In some meetings, they discuss the particular effects of alcohol and drug use on family and daily life. This discussion is also an opportunity for Lisa to express her feelings and fears, and discuss the support provided by child protection services.

The multi-professional team will decide with Lisa and Steve how best to continue working with their family. The team will estimate the support that will benefit Steve and the family most and make plans accordingly. Possibilities are, for example, rehabilitation in institutional care or open care; couple, family, and individual therapy; network meetings with child protection services; and participation in peer or self-help groups. The social worker's role with the family depends partly on her/his supplementary education. The qualification required to be recognized as a legal social worker is a Master's degree in social work. However, many have schooled themselves as some kind of legalized therapist. The professional title for an A-clinic social worker is "social therapist."

Case study #3

Substance-abusing Street Children

BY TUMANI MALINGA-MUSAMBA FROM BOTSWANA

Ben is a 14-year-old boy who is HIV positive and does not adhere to his antiretroviral (ARV) treatment. His CD4 count has dropped from thousands to less than 500. He is an orphan and was born HIV positive. His mother died of AIDS when he was five years old. He was an only child and has never known his father. Since the death of his mother, his maternal grandmother has been his guardian. This grandmother is in her late 60s and also struggles with medical conditions. She is responsible for Ben's health and welfare and also takes care of five other orphaned children in the family aged between seven and 15 years.

Ben's grandmother benefits from the state welfare program where she is registered under the destitute policy. In addition, all the orphans under her care are registered under the government orphan care program whereby each receives monthly food assistance. The family has no other source of financial support.

Even though he had been attending and doing well in school, Ben started missing classes and his grades began to drop when he was in his fifth year at primary school. Days would go by with his whereabouts being unknown by his grandmother. These behaviors impacted not only his school performance, but also his medication adherence. He has not been to school for the past two years.

Ben's grandmother reports that when he started running away, she would look for him in the community and was unable to find him. She states that, at times, community members inform her that he has been seen at the bus station, market, or shops where he is asking for money to buy food. Community members also tell Ben's grandmother that he has been seen sniffing glue. Whenever Ben's grandmother looks for him, she cannot find him. She therefore suspects that whenever Ben sees her, he will hide. His cousins report that they always see him in the community, and that he sometimes comes home when his grandmother is not in. Generally, Ben does not want to listen to or take orders from his grandmother and she is concerned about his health and well-being.

Recently, Ben was referred to a social worker by his doctor who reported concern since the patient's CD4 count had been dropping drastically over the past year. During the first meeting with the social workers, for the first time Ben said that he did not want to stay where there are rules and regulations, and he did not want to take his medication. In addition, he said that his grandmother wanted him to bathe regularly and go to school, but that he is not interested in doing those things. Ben seemed knowledgeable about why he should take his medication and the effects of medication non-adherence.

Substance-abusing Street Children: A Social Worker from El Salvador Responds

BY RENÉ OLATE & WILSON ALVARADO FROM EL SALVADOR

Prevalence and Incidence

Delinquency is one of the most significant problems in the Latin American region nowadays. According to a regional assessment of the crucial issues facing the region, delinquency has been identified as the primary problem, for the first time exceeding other problems such as unemployment, economic problems, and poverty (Latinobarómetro, 2011). A standard indicator employed to analyze levels of violence and delinquency is the homicide rate per 100,000 people. Three countries in Latin America display alarming figures using this indicator: El Salvador, Guatemala, and Honduras. These countries are referred to as the "Northern Triangle of Violence" (Aguilar, 2007). According to the United Nations Development Program (UNDP, 2009), the average homicide rate for these countries was 53 per 100,000 people, more than double the average of the entire region and extremely high compared to Argentina, Uruguay, and Chile, with rates of 5, 4 and 1 respectively. The cost of criminal violence in El Salvador in 2003 was US $1.7 billion, approximately 12% of the GDP (World Bank, 2011).

Violence and delinquency in El Salvador are associated with the following factors: civil war, a culture of violence, disorganized urban development, poverty, lack of opportunities for youth, marginalization, and the transit of drugs from South America to Mexico and the US (Cruz, 2007). However, one of the most cited contributors to the situation of violence and delinquency in the Northern Triangle is the presence of transnational youth gangs, with two main clusters in particular: Mara Salvatrucha (MS-13) and Eighteenth Street (*Barrio 18*) (Cruz, 2007). Both gangs originated in poor communities in Los Angeles, California. Eighteenth Street was established by primarily Mexican immigrants in the 1960s and Mara Salvatrucha by Salvadoran immigrants escaping from the civil war in the 1980s (Savenije, 2009). Many of the youth gang members, documented and undocumented, were deported from the US for various crimes in the 1990s and during the first decade of this century, bringing with them the American youth gang culture (Seelke, 2011).

This new, imported gang culture, combined with issues of poverty, social exclusion, a culture of violence, the availability of drugs, family problems, and difficulties of youth in defining individual identity are the most important factors associated with the phenomenon of youth gangs (Cruz, 2010). The number of youth who belong to gangs in El Salvador is debated. For the Northern Triangle, different accounts estimate between 70,000 and 300,000 youth gang members. Conservative estimates in El Salvador suggest that there are over 20,000, with more than 8,500 in prison in 2010. Police statistics for the years 2009 and 2010 identified that gangs were involved in 22–33% of all homicides and extortion in the country. These official numbers confirm the assumption that youth gangs are only a factor in the context of violence and delinquency in El Salvador.

Country Policies

The government's response to the problem of violence and delinquency has been generally characterized by suppression, also known as the "iron fist" ("*Mano Dura*") approach. These policies are based on the deterrence criminology theory, which argues that an increase in penalties results in a decrease in crime. Several types of "Mano Dura" legislation have been enacted, mainly in El Salvador. Unfortunately, the results of these punitive policies have been very limited (Aguilar, 2006). Furthermore, some researchers claim that these policies have had numerous unintended consequences (Savenije, 2009). Indeed, during the implementation of these policies, the number of homicides and crime in general increased in the Northern Triangle (UNDP, 2009).

Despite the formal inclusion of components related to prevention and intervention at the community level, "Mano Dura" policies are heavily oriented to suppression and punishment (Klein & Maxson, 2006). The emphasis of these policies is rooted in a police and control perspective (Howell, 2009). For youth, this legislation has a very simple message: "lock them up". In addition to being ineffective in reducing the overall crime in Salvadoran society, the net effects of these policies are the criminalization of youth living in poor communities and the overcrowding of prisons (Olate & Salas-Wrigth, 2010). There are also several social government and NGOs programs emphasizing the prevention of risky behavior among youth. However, these programs are not targeting the high-risk group of youth in communities with active gang members.

Equipo Nahual, an NGO working with high risk youth and youth gang members, emphasizes harm reduction and youth development through activities for youth. Professionals working for this organization include social workers, psychologists, and lawyers. The social workers are street-workers, involved in mediation on the dangerous street corners of the most marginalized communities in San Salvador. In addition, social workers organize job workshops as well as sports and recreational activities for youth. The job trainings include carpentry, baking, silk screen printing, and sewing.

Complementing the job training, *Equipo Nahual* offers psychosocial workshops in human relations and conflict resolution. Social workers run the psychosocial activities while a local carpenter or baker teaches specific technical vocational knowledge and skills. In addition, social workers provide counseling and case management to the youth participating in the workshops. In prisons, social workers support the rehabilitation process of incarcerated youth. The social workers are also involved in evaluation and research through a longitudinal study of high-risk youth behaviors and interventions (Olate, Salas-Wright, & Vaughn, 2011).

It is through social workers' presence on the streets that they are able to engage and begin to build rapport with high risk youth and youth involved in gangs. Since policies based on repression and punishment have failed, *Equipo Nahual* has implemented social work community prevention and intervention strategies for marginalized youth based on the public health perspective and solidarity approach. *Equipo Nahual* understands that youth are not only the main perpetrators of violence, but also the main victims. This organization emphasizes that youth violence is the most visible phenomenon of a violent society surrounded by multiple social problems, such as alcoholism, drug addiction and drug trafficking, a lack of opportunities, and a deficient delivery of public education and health services (Alvarado, 2010).

A Social Worker Responds

Though Ben is not gang involved, he is struggling with issues that are quite common among the youth that Equipo Nahual serves. Ben has medical and psychosocial problems. He is a 14-year-old adolescent who a) is HIV positive, b) dropped out of school, c) is using drugs, and d) is a runaway. Ben is living in the context of poverty and social, physical, and psychological vulnerability. Considering Ben's unique situation, the objectives of a social work intervention would be related to four main issues: 1) the urgent need for medication adherence for his HIV treatment, 2) the need to overcome drug use and probable addiction, and 3) the need for social reintegration both at school and in his grandmother's home.

The first objective would be that Ben regularly takes his HIV medication, particularly now that his glycoproteins CD4 have significantly dropped. US guidelines advocate treatment when an individual's CD4 cell count falls under 500 cells/mm^3. Starting therapy at higher CD4 cell counts reduced the risk of AIDS-related illnesses or death. Linking Ben to local health services would be fundamental in order to accomplish this goal. It is also important that Ben realizes that he is not alone in his experience of having HIV; there are many people his age who also suffer from this virus. Encouraging Ben to participate in a support group with other HIV positive youth is very important. By joining a support group, he could not only reflect upon his situation and feelings, but he could also have the experience of being supported by others his age.

The second objective would be to quit or reduce his drug consumption. The abuse of glue is generally associated with the consumption of marijuana and many other drugs. The low cost and easy access to glue often causes it to be the drug of choice among marginalized youth. In this case, it would be important to glean the degree and frequency of Ben's use of drugs, as well as a list of the drugs he has been using on a regular basis. This would provide the information necessary to determine whether or not he would need to be admitted to a detoxification and drug rehabilitation program.

Connecting Ben to a drug treatment and rehabilitation program would not be an easy intervention given the limited public services available and the high demand for drug treatment in El Salvador. In addition, the objective of complete abstinence from drugs in a poor community in San Salvador is very difficult to achieve, thus perhaps having a goal of gradual reduction of drug consumption might be a more realistic approach. Harm reduction aligns with the service philosophy that social workers at *Equipo Nahual* currently employ.

The third objective is to help Ben reintegrate both in his school environment and at home with his family. His grandmother appears to be a person who is concerned about Ben's situation. She has left home many times in search of him. It seems that Ben, wishing to avoid following the house rules, rejects his grandmother. Reviving and nurturing this relationship is fundamental. The social worker should begin by working to build rapport with Ben's grandmother. It would be helpful to explore Ben's grandmother's philosophy around child rearing, particularly that of establishing and enforcing rules, communication, and discipline. It is likely that Ben's grandmother is in need of significant support, particularly given the complex challenges presented by Ben and potentially by the other children in her care.

The social worker might assess the need to connect Ben's grandmother to other additional resources and supports in the community. The social worker should also provide individual therapy with Ben, as long as Ben understands that the therapy session will be canceled if he arrives high. With Ben, the social worker might help explore and work on how his past traumas and losses affect his choices today. The social worker might help Ben develop constructive coping skills and improve his self-care, particularly regarding his HIV treatment. Ultimately, family therapy would be very useful. This could begin with meetings between Ben and his grandmother, to work on improving communication, and understanding and strengthening respect. The family therapy may then expand to incorporate the other children living in the home, if deemed useful and if Ben agrees. The therapy sessions could be provided collaboratively with psychologists.

The goal of returning to either regular school or to a school specializing in providing services to drop-outs is a priority. It seems that Ben is capable of being a good student and would be able to complete the equivalent of a high school diploma. Perhaps he might even aspire to attend college, with the help of social work interventions, and family and community support.

The stated objectives are based on a wraparound perspective, wherein multiple agencies and professionals coordinate services and collaboratively implement diverse interventions. Attempting to accomplish these three objectives would be a difficult and demanding task. Limited resources in Salvadoran public social service organizations and NGOs would be a key obstacle potentially thwarting the success of the suggested interventions.

Ben's path to social rehabilitation and medical treatment is likely to be arduous and somewhat cyclical; the chances of Ben relapsing are high. The commitment of NGOs and local public agencies would be fundamentally important. The social workers at *Equipo Nahual* provide accompaniment, follow up, acceptance, and understanding; all of which Ben desperately needs. Based on a collective effort involving his family, the local school, professionals at public organizations, NGOs and the community, it would be possible for Ben to achieve success and begin to envision a brighter future.

The core values of *Equipo Nahual* social work interventions focus on the understanding of human relations within the broader context of community social participation and deliberation processes. This organization pursues the reconstruction of broken social fabric through participation in workshops and circles of reconciliation. The key characteristics of these methodologies, which emphasize a restorative or reparative perspective of justice, are: the belief that there are possibilities for repentance and forgiveness, the acknowledgement of both victims and offenders' roles and rights within a whole context (social, economic, political, and cultural), and the focus on the community as a facilitator of restoration, reconciliation, and healing (Alvarado, 2010). For *Equipo Nahual*, these are more than methodologies; it is an ethical framework for living and working in marginalized communities.

Substance-abusing Street Children: A Social Worker from the US Responds

BY DARSELL M. HARRIS

Prevalence and Incidence

The number of homeless people in the US is believed to be between 600,000 and 2.5 million. Within this group, it is estimated that youth make up 5 per cent of the total (Congressional Research Services [CRS], 2005. Unfortunately, the use of drugs and other substances is very common among street children. Twenty-five to 90 per cent of street children use drugs, and it appears that those in the US are particularly hooked on crack cocaine (WHO, 2000). In 2009, the Substance Abuse and Mental Health Services Administration (SAMHSA) survey revealed that 61 per cent of 12—17-year-olds abused banned drugs, and the rate of alcohol abuse was 4.6 per cent (SAMHSA, 2010). In the same year, a survey suggested that, among 1.9 million youths who experienced major depressive disorders,

19.9 per cent were victims of substance use disorders (SAMHSA, 2012). However, statistics from surveys may not reflect the incidence of substance use and abuse among homeless youth (Parriott & Auerswald, 2009; Slesnick, Meyers, Meade & Segelken, 2000). For instance, in a nationally representative survey comparing youth from the street, shelters, and the National Household Survey on Drug Abuse (NHSDA), researchers found that the prevalence of substance use for street children was higher than for all the other groups. Of the 12 substances that were measured, 71 per cent of the street youth, 46 per cent of the shelter youth, and 25 per cent of the NHSDA youth had used three or more substances. Thirty-five per cent of street youth, 13 per cent of youth in shelters, and 4 per cent of youth from the NHSDA had used six or more substances. Street youth had the highest mean for the number of substances used with 4.6 substances, followed by shelter youth with 2.2, and youth from the NHSDA at 1.7 (Greene, Ennett & Ringwalt, 1997).

Country Policies

In the last quarter of the twentieth century, the social work profession's predominating agenda involved professionalizing the field with psycho-logically-based interventions (Cox, 2001). Social work became defined as direct, individual practice in the form of aid to individual clients and families with targeted material assistance or interventions using the diagnostic and statistical manual of mental diseases DSM-IV. The National Association of Social Workers (NASW, 2005) defines social work as a helping profession in which individuals, groups, and/or communities are assisted by social workers to enhance or restore their capacity to function socially. Currently, social workers are active in all areas of society, providing a valuable resource for those who are distressed, disadvantaged, or vulnerable.

It is important to understand the role of social workers who operate within the context of the child welfare system in the US. This role contributes to a negative view of social work since child welfare authorities can remove abused or neglected children from the custody of parents. Child welfare is a term used to describe a set of government services designed to protect children and encourage family stability. These services typically include investigation of alleged child abuse and neglect ("protective services" or "family preservation services"). The idea behind child welfare programs is that, in certain circumstances, the interests of the child could be better served by removing children from the care of their parents and placing them in state custody. While a preferred scenario is to support the family while keeping it intact, the circumstances may be too severe for the child.

Under these conditions, children are removed on a temporary basis while the parents, and possibly siblings, receive supportive services until the family is deemed to be in a position to resume care of the child.

A Social Worker Responds

Ben is a high risk multi-problem child who is engaging in dangerous problematic behaviors. His runaway behavior negates a social worker's option of providing in-home services for him and his family. In review of his offenses of truancy, incorrigibility, and ungovernability, Ben is likely to enter the child welfare system as a dependent child. For example, the Pennsylvania Juvenile Act defines a person under the age of 18 as "dependent" if he/she has committed a specific act or acts of habitual disobedience of the reasonable and lawful commands of his/her parent, guardian or other custodian and who is ungovernable and found to be in need of care, treatment, or while subject to compulsory school attendance is habitually and without justification truant from school. The child welfare system is the government agency that is responsible for taking care of children when their parents are unable to care for them. In Pennsylvania, the state child welfare system is called the Office of Children, Youth and Families and is within the Department of Public Welfare. Ben's actions warrant his removal from his grandmother's home and placement in protective custody under a time-limited voluntary agreement. His removal from the home requires an adjudication hearing.

It should be noted that Ben is currently in a kinship placement, living with his grandmother since he is an orphan. Kinship caretakers are typically the least restrictive placement options and can preserve the child's connections to family. Kinship placement considerations include geographical proximity to the family and community, educational stability, and cultural relevance of the placement to assure permanence and well-being. Returning Ben to his grandmother would be the eventual goal of a social worker since there is no evidence to suggest that she is unable to care for her grandchildren. Although it is noted that the family is living in poverty, there is no indication that Ben's grandmother lacks appropriate parenting skills. However, upon Ben's return home, additional in-home services would be made available to her at her request.

After the adjudication hearing, Ben will be placed in a residential treatment facility (RTF). Residential treatment facilities are childcare facilities that are licensed under Chapter 3810 of 55 PA Code that provide 24-hour living arrangements and mental health treatment for children and adolescents in need of structured and therapeutic intervention (Value

Options, 2011). Children placed in an RTF setting are found to be experiencing social, behavioral, educational and/or emotional problems, and are unable to function successfully in their home or their community. Placement is focused on treatment with the hope that the child can transition back to the family or community care as soon as possible.

A psychiatric evaluation for authorization of the RTF admission is performed by a licensed psychologist who must recommend why this level of care is medically necessary and why less intensive, less restrictive services are not expected to adequately meet the identified needs of the child. The treatment standards for residential treatment facilities that Ben will participate in are (Value Options, 2011, p. 9):

- Milieu therapy: the therapeutic environment is expected to provide regular opportunities for treatment and therapeutic activities;
- Individual therapy: every child is expected to be provided with the opportunity for weekly scheduled one-on-one interaction with a Master's level clinician and spontaneous individual therapy opportunities for intervention;
- Family therapy: each child is expected to participate in family-focused therapy sessions on at least a weekly basis;
- Opportunities for therapeutic leave: this option is very effective in helping children and their family prepare for discharge from the setting;
- Group therapy: this core component of daily programming focuses on anger management, self-awareness, social skill development, developing positive relationships with peers and family, conflict resolution, and anxiety management. Specialized groups such as substance abuse and HIV education are offered when needed;
- Skill building opportunities within the residential treatment facility and community settings;
- Opportunities for community participation on a weekly basis;
- Medication administration and monitoring on a daily basis and at least monthly monitoring by a psychiatrist and physician.

Residential treatment is not intended to fix the child, but rather is an intervention to stabilize the child and promote successful community reintegration. Upon completion of the above outlined service plan, it is expected that Ben will be able to return home to his grandmother and require minimal supervision.

Exercises

In class

The following topics, for in-class discussion, should be explored in an atmosphere of respect and acceptance of difference. In this way, a better understanding and conceptualization of the issues will be obtained.

- How would you as a social worker respond to one of the cases presented in this chapter? Describe why your response would be different from or similar to those provided.
- Consideration should be given to law enforcement agencies and their role in cases involving illicit substance use and abuse. Do these agencies coordinate efforts in regard to substance abuse in your home country?
- To what extent do the most marginalized social groups engage in substance abuse? If you have ascertained that they do, how is this reflected in their lifestyles and challenges faced by them?

Out of class

For each of the exercises below, select a country different from your home country and the countries discussed in this chapter and present your findings on that society to your peers in class.

- Search for sources of information in another country on substance abuse and summarize resources for addressing the issue.
- Consider the laws on substance abuse in another country and compare them to legislation in your home country.
- Conduct a literature review of substance abuse in one or two countries and extract the salient issues emerging from the research.
- Develop a list of agencies (state, NGO, and community or faith-based organizations) that assist in cases of substance abuse. What are their mission statements, and to what extent are social workers involved "at the rockface?"
- Interview two social workers about their knowledge of substance abuse in their own (or another) country. Explore their views regarding community attitudes and incidence of the problem.

References

Adoption of Children Act 1952, Bechuanaland/Botswana. No. 28:01.

Aguilar, J. (2006). "The counterproductive effects of Iron Fist plans." *Revista de Pensamiento Iberoamericano*, 16, 81–94.

—. (2007). *The youth gangs or maras in the northern triangle of Central America.* San Salvador: UCA Editores

Alvarado, W. (2010). "Youth and violence: The meaning of an open perspective about the results in social participation." Unpublished manuscript.

Andrade, L. Walters, E. E., Gentil, V., & Laurenti, R. (2002). "Prevalence of ICD-10 Mental disorders in a catchment area in the city of São Paulo, Brazil." *Social Psychiatry and Psychiatric Epidemiology*, 37, 316–25.

Asuni, T., & Pela, O. (1986). "Drug abuse in Africa." *Bulletin on Narcotics*, 38, 55–64. Retrieved from http://www.unodc.org/unodc/en/data-and-analysis/bulletin/bulletin_1986-01-01_1_page007.html

Baron, S. W. (1999). "Street youths and substance use: The role of background, street lifestyle, and economic factors." *Youth & Society*, 31 (1), 3–26.

Child and Adolescent Treaty 1990 (b) Brazil. No. 8.069

Cox, A.L. (2001). "BSW students favor strengths/empowerment-based generalist practice." *Families in Society*, 82 (3), 305–13.

Cruz, J.M. (Ed.) (2007). *Street gangs in Central America.* San Salvador: UCA Editores.

Cruz, J.M. (2010). Central American maras: From youth street gangs to transnational protection rackets. *Global Crime, 11*(4), 379–98.

Fals-Stewart, W., Birchler, G. R., & O'Farrell, T. J. (1999). Drug-abusing patients and their intimate partners: Dyadic adjustment, relationship stability, and substance use. *Journal of Abnormal Psychology*, 108 (1), 11–23.

Forsell, M., Virtanen, A., Jääskeläinen, M., Alho, H., & Partanen, A. (2010). *Finland – Drug Situation 2010. National Report to the EMCDDA.* Helsinki: National Institute for Health and Welfare.

Granfelt, R. (1993). "Psychosocial orientation in social work." In R. Granfelt, H. Jokiranta, S. Karvinen, A.-L. Matthies, & A. Pohjola (Eds.) *Monisärmäinen sosiaalityö* (pp. 175–227). Helsinki: Sosiaaliturvan Keskusliitto.

Greene, J. M., Ennett, S. T., & Ringwalt, C. L. (1997). "Substance use among runaway and homeless youth in three national samples." *American Journal Of Public Health*, 87 (2), 229–35.

Hakkarainen, P., & Metso, L. (2005). "Wet high and year 2004." *Yhteiskuntapolitiikka*, 3 (70), 252–65.

Hasin, D. S., Stinson, F. S., Ogburn, E., & Grant, B. F. (2007). "Prevalence, correlates, disability, and comorbidity of DSM-IV alcohol abuse and dependence in the United States: Results from the National Epidemiological Survey on Alcohol and Related Conditions." *Archives of General Psychiatry*, 64 (7), 830.

Hawkins, J. D., Catalano, R. F., & Miller, J. Y. (1992). "Risk and protective factors for alcohol and other drug problems in adolescence and early adulthood:

Implications for substance abuse prevention." *Psychological Bulletin*, 112 (1), 64–105.

Health Organic Law 1990 (a) Brazil. No. 8.080

Holmila, M. (2001). "Family, intoxicants and gender." *Yhteiskuntapolitiikka*, 1 (66), 55–61.

Howell, J. C. (2009). *Preventing and reducing juvenile delinquency: A comprehensive framework* (2nd edn). Thousand Oaks, CA: Sage.

Kainulainen, H. (2009). "Intoxicant and dopecrimes 2009." In: *Rikollisuustilanne 2009. Tutkimuksia 250*. Helsinki: Oikeuspoliittinen Tutkimuslaitos. Retrieved from http://www.optula.om.fi/1284990230726

Klein, M., & Maxson, C. (2006). *Street gang patterns and policies*. New York: Oxford University Press.

Kuusisto, K. (2009). "Different routes for recovering from substance abuse." In T. Tammi, M. Aalto, & A. Koski-Jännes, (Eds.) *Irti Päihdeongelmasta*. (pp. 32–48). Helsinki: Edita.

Latinobarómetro (2011). *Annual Report 2010*. Santiago, Chile: Latinobarómetro.

Mäkelä, P., Mustonen, H., & Christoffer, T. (2010). "*Finland drinks. Alcohol use and it´s changes 1968–2008 among Finnish Population*. Helsinki: Terveyden ja hyvinvoinnin laitos. Retrieved from http://www.thl.fi.thl-client/pdfs/371e1e08-9bc1-47ea-81aa-68b04f27088c

Miller, W. R., & Rollnick, S. (2002). *Motivational interviewing: Preparing people for change*. New York: The Guilford Press.

Ministry of Health and Social Welfare of Korea (2011). *National Health Plan 2020*.

Mönkkönen, K. (2007). *Interaction. Dialogical client work*. Helsinki: Edita.

National Institute for Health and Welfare (Finland). (2009). "Alcoholic beverage consumption." Retrieved from http://stakes.fi/tilastot/tilastotie-dotteet/2010/Tr10_.pdf

Olate, R., & Salas-Wright, C. (2010). "How to intervene in the problems of youth violence and delinquency?" *Revista de Trabajo Social*, 79, 7–21.

Olate, R., Salas-Wright, C., & Vaughn, M. (2011). "A cross-national comparison of externalizing behaviors among high risk youth and youth gang members in metropolitan Boston and San Salvador." *Victims & Offenders*, 6 (4), 356–69.

Päihdelinkki (2011b). *Outpatient services in Finland*. Retrieved from http://www.paihdelinkki.fi/foreinger-info/in-treament

Parriott, A. M., & Auerswald, C. L. (2009). "Incidence and predictors of onset of injection drug use in a San Francisco cohort of homeless youth." *Substance Use & Misuse*, 44 (13), 1958–970.

Psychiatric Reform Law 2001 Brazil. No. 10.216

Room, R., Babor, T., & Rehm, J. (2005). "Alcohol and public health." *The Lancet*, 365 (9458), 519–30.

Savenije, W. (2009). *Maras and schoolgangs: Gangs and youth violence in the marginal communities of Central America*. San Salvador: FLACSO Programa El Salvador.

Schmidt, M. I., Duncan, B. B., Silva, G. A., Menezes, A. M., Monteiro, C. A.,

Barreto, S. M., Chor, D., & Menezes, P. R. (2011). "Chronic non-communicable diseases in Brazil: Burden and current challenges", *The Lancet – Health in Brazil 4*. Retrieved from DOI10.1016/SO140-6736(11)60135-9

Schober, R., & Annis, H. M. (1996). "Barriers to help-seeking for change in drinking: a gender-focused review of the literature." *Addictive Behaviors*, 21 (1), 81–92.

Seelke, R. C. (2011). *Gangs in Central America*. Congressional Research Service. Washington, D.C: The Library of Congress.

Seikkula, J., & Arnkil, T. E. (2006). *Dialogical work with social networks*. Helsinki: Kustannusosakeyhtiö Tammi.

Senad (2005). *II Home survey on psychotropic drug use in Brazil*. Sao Paulo:Pagina e Grafica Editora e Letras.

Shin, M. S. (2002). "Problem drinking and related factors among adults in Korea." *The Journal of Korean Alcohol Science*, 3 (1), 111–30.

Slesnick, N., Meyers, R., Meade, M., & Segelken, D. (2000). "Bleak and hopeless no more. Engagement of reluctant substance-abusing runaway youth and their families." *Journal of substance Abuse Treatment*, 19 (3), 215–22.

Substance Abuse and Mental Health Services Administration (SAMHSA) Office of Applied Studies. 2010. *Results from the 2009 National Survey on Drug Use and Health: Volume I. Summary of National Findings*. Rockville, MD: United States Department of Health and Human Services.

Substance Abuse and Mental Health Services Administration (SAMHSA) Office of Applied Studies. 2012. *Results from the 2010 National Survey on Drug Use and Health: Volume I. Summary of National Findings*. Rockville, MD: United States Department of Health and Human Services.

Willis, J. (2006). "Drinking crisis? Change and continuity in cultures of drinking in sub-Saharan Africa." *African Journal of Drug and Alcohol Studies*, 5, 1–16.

Woods, M. E., & Robinson, H. (1996). "Psychosocial theory and social work treatment." In F. Turner (Ed.) *Social work treatment; Interlocking theoretical approaches* (pp. 555–80). New York: The Free Press.

World Health Organization (WHO). (2000) "Working with street children. Module 3: Understanding substance use among street children – A training package on substance use, sexual and reproductive health including HIV/AIDS and STDs." Geneva: WHO Retrived from. http://whqlibdoc.who.int/hq/2000/WHO_MSD_MDP_00.14_Module3.pdf

World Health Organization (WHO). (2011). *Global status report on alcohol and health*. Geneva: WHO.

Yoon, M. S. (2010). "The current situation and developmental direction of Korean addiction service delivery system." *Mental Health and Social Work*, 35, 234–66.

<table>
<tr><td>**10**</td><td></td></tr>
</table>

Concluding Remarks

By Caren J. Frost and Isaac Karikari

As we read the case studies and analyses for this book, we were struck by the range of practices in the field of international social work. This recognition is important because, as Akimoto (2007) noted, "We need to understand social work more in an international context." The practices discussed by the authors of these studies are diverse and more clearly defined based on the length of time social work has been a profession in the cultural, political, legal, and economic landscape of each country presented here. The professional training of the social workers writing for this book illustrates the different cultural and educational milieus in which social work has developed. According to the IFSW definition of social work[1], interventions should utilize theories about social systems and human behavior. These cases and analyses address such theories in their own country contexts, and provide us with a better understanding about how social problems are defined and acted on by the professionals working in these systems. A brief consideration of the similarities and differences in social work will enable us to see the connections among social work practices at a global level.

Similarities in Social Work Professionalism

There are commonalities in social work, notably in the areas of education, practice, and research (Gray & Fook, 2004). Cross-cultural influence in the development of social work dates back to the late-nineteenth and early-twentieth centuries (Kniephoff-Knebel & Seibel, 2008). With the increase

---

1 The social work profession promotes social change, problem-solving in human relationships, and the empowerment and liberation of people to enhance well-being. Utilizing theories of human behavior and social systems, social work intervenes at the points where people interact with their environments. Principles of human rights and social justice are fundamental to social work (IFSW, 2000).

in international social work research, it has become evident that similar social problems are prevalent all over the globe (Hendriks et al., 2008; Lalayants, Tripodi & Jung, 2009). How social work is viewed as a profession and occupation impacts the design and delivery of social service interventions for people in need. Across all nations where social work has a presence, the empowerment of people is a theme central to professional processes and practice (Hare, 2004); this theme is very clear in the case analyses from each of the countries represented.

Common to practitioners in different countries is the development of professional organizations and the formation of associations. However, in Botswana and South Africa (Weiss-Gal & Welbourne, 2008), national associations for practitioners are just being founded. In other countries where there are no official professional organizations, social workers utilize the IFSW standards as the basis for their practice, which is not ideal since these standards are not culture/country specific; however, these IFSW standards provide a common foundation for understanding the values associated with social work.

On the other hand, in India, Sweden, the US, the UK, Hungary, Spain, Germany, and Ghana, such professional associations exist and are quite active with regular conferences, workshops, and so on available to association members (Kreitzer & Wilson, 2010; Weiss-Gal & Welbourne, 2008). These associations and organizations provide standards and consistency in understanding how to construct social work interventions. They also allow for a forum for members to meet, explore, and review how social work should be practiced. Associations and organizations highlight the professionalism of the occupation of social work, which in many countries is an issue that hinders comprehensive practice and service delivery. In addition, not only does a professional organization add to the status of a professional, it also provides information about ethical and current practices for social workers.

Professional social work associations and organizations have specific values that they promote for their members to consider when working at the micro, mezzo, and macro levels. For example, the National Association of Social Workers (NASW), the umbrella organization for social work professionals in the US, states its core values as "service, social justice, dignity and worth of the person, importance of human relationships, integrity and competence" (NASW, 2008, "Preamble"). The five basic values stated in the British Association of Social Workers (BASW) code of ethics are "human dignity and worth, social justice, service to humanity, integrity and competence" (BASW, 2001, p. 2). The code of ethics of the BASW shares common elements with the code of ethics of its US counterpart (Lindsey, 2005) since both espouse a commitment to social justice, a belief in human dignity, and a common stance against discrimination (Lindsey, 2005). The values for both these large organizations are linked to the UN Declaration of Human Rights, which provides the Western lens about human rights and how social justice is constructed.

In the US and the UK, practice at the micro level, such as direct practice with individuals and families, is what most social workers provide. Social workers' involvement in macro practice appears to be secondary (Weiss, 2006). Similar to the US and the UK, countries like Hungary have codified guidelines for ethical social work practice. Germany, Sweden, and Spain have social work codes of ethics based on the principles and standards of the IFSW (Weiss-Gal & Welbourne, 2008). Using the IFSW standards may indeed promote an inequality of understanding about the cultural context of the human condition (Akimoto, 2007). Thus a more thorough consideration of international social work practice, as set forth in this book, is crucial to delineate country landscapes for a clearer context to emerge.

Differences in Social Work Practices and Parameters

International exchanges and collaborations in social work practice are not a novelty. Italian social work, for instance, owes its development partly to knowledge and experiences gleaned from other nations, particularly social work practice in the US (Fargion, 2008). However, social workers are divided on the issue of the universal application of social work values (Leung, 2007; Midgley, 2001). Some believe that these standards constitute a reflection of Western models and practices that do not fit other cultures and are therefore suggestive of attempts to impose one culture on another (Parrot, 2009). Cultural values influence the nature of policies and actual social work practice (Lindsey, 2005). Cultural tensions often occur when practitioners attempt to apply social work values and ethics rooted in Western traditions and culture in non-Western cultures. A conflict occurs because of the poor fit between professional tenets and cultural and ethnic values (Akimoto, 2007; Miu Chung, 2008).

In countries such as China and Taiwan, the political climate, as well as cultural norms, affect social work practice. Social work values such as individual justice, independence, freedom, and self-determination, which are integral aspects of Western social work, go against the basic ideals of some cultures (Toseland & McClive-Reed, 2009). In India, discussions around diversity are not a dominant feature in social work practice as they are in the US. Certain issues relating to diversity are unsuitable for discussion in Indian classrooms (Kohli & Faul, 2005). In Zimbabwe, social workers do not undertake personal initiative in their social work practice—they implement government policies only (Moldovan & Moyo, 2007).

The Japanese situation is similar. Content on cultural and ethnic diversity have not featured prominently in social work education in Japan (Saito & Johns, 2009); however, with the recent influx of foreign health care workers into Japan, these discussions are beginning. Further, in Japan the use of concepts such as empowerment, informed consent, and advocacy is common, but they do not form the basis for social work practice.

Another important difference in social work practice that exists is how different social work contexts use words differently. In welfare states such as the UK, the words "needs" and "wants" hold different meanings; however, in Japan the two are synonymous (Saito & Johns, 2009). These cultural, political, and linguistic differences are worth noting, because, as illustrated in the case studies and analyses in this book, they all have implications regarding practice in the international arena (Saito & Johns, 2009).

Religious and spiritual beliefs, as well as regional culture, influence the application of interventions in practice (Stewart & Koeske, 2006). In much the same way, students' and practitioners' attitudes are very much influenced by the social climate of the societies and countries where they practice (Kohli & Faul, 2005). In one instance a social worker encountered a conflicting situation between his professional values and the cultural values. The worker had an unmarried but pregnant Muslim client who, just like the worker, was a Bedouin-Arab. Bedouin-Arabs are an Arabic speaking people of the Middle East. Within the Bedouin culture, the same culture in which he practiced as a social worker, to be unmarried and pregnant calls for the punishment of death, which is a common punishment for women caught in premarital and extramarital affairs (Al-Krenawi, 1999). Regarding the conflict and the personal dilemma he faced, the social worker wrote:

> Being familiar with both the cultural and social work profession values and canons, this led to a struggle within me—as a Bedouin-Arab whose values had been derived from the cultural/religious values and customs of my tribe and as a social worker trained to follow professional values derived from Western-oriented formal theory and knowledge. On one hand, I was trained to respect the client and treat her with empathy and support. On the other hand, all of my background demanded that I function within the cultural context within which I had been reared (Al-Krenawi, 1999, p. 490).

Further, variations exist in child welfare policies and protection structures in different countries (Dubowitz, 2009). In a study on child-centered social work practice in Australia, Canada, and Sweden, researchers found that structural as well as contextual factors are important for determining the models adopted for practice with children (Rasmusson, Hyvönen, Nygren & Khoo, 2010). In Australian child welfare practice, effort is made toward maintaining a balance between meeting the needs of children and making them active participants of the process, seeking their views in offering them care (referred to as a rights-based approach). In contrast to this, Canada is more inclined toward needs, and Sweden more toward rights (Rasmusson et al., 2010). As noted in the case studies and analyses in this book, these country and cultural differences allow us a more concrete understanding of the cultural, political, and economic backdrops within which social work in practiced in the countries represented in the writings.

Throughout the book, one sees that social work as a profession grapples with the concept of cultural relativity. This concept in anthropology and social work is connected to the idea that a professional starts where the participant and/or client is. For most of the analyses in this book, social workers are attempting to provide ideas about culturally relative and culturally appropriate practice; however, in some countries the religious, cultural, and political parameters make being culturally relative very difficult. For example, in the case analysis about homosexuality in Ghana, it is apparent that religious and cultural pressures dictate how a person who identifies as a homosexual will be treated—homosexuality is illegal in Ghana, and so a social worker begins with that premise in providing social services.

Summary Thoughts

In this book, there are a number of issues that we do not address. For example, lacking are discussions related to disabilities, physical health, occupational health, social justice, and gender issues. There are many additional areas that could and should be explored through the international lens of social work; however, lack of space prohibited us from doing so.

In order to determine the prevalence, incidence, and country policies of the problems presented in the book, individual authors had to research and provide a pertinent summary of this information. These data are often not available for a country; as a consequence, some of the sections are quite brief on these issues. For countries where social work has been established for a longer period of time, more is known about the prevalence and incidence of the social problems and countries policies are more clearly defined. Having these pieces of information readily at hand aids social workers in better serving clients and vulnerable populations in their countries. Readers will notice significant variation in the specificity of these sections of each case analysis, due to the reasons detailed above.

Some of the fascinating discussions in this book connect to what constitutes legal age for a variety of activities, concepts linked to property ownership, and cultural ideas around types of marriages, women's and men's roles, the role of children, and so on. Descriptions about these cultural parameters add to the complexity of social work practice in these cross-cultural settings and provide depth to any analysis that can be conducted about social work practice.

This book makes clear that we need to invest more in terms of sharing information about practice and social service design, implementation, and delivery across countries and contexts. Questions about how practice is developed, professionalized, and standardized need to be asked and answered at local, regional, and global levels. Without a more regular exchange of ideas, social work practitioners will not be as empowered or knowledgeable about how to promote social change and assist in solving human problems which are the premise of international social work.

References

Akimoto, T. (2007). "Brief note: The unipolar world and inequality in social work: A response to James Midgley, 'Global inequality, power and the unipolar world: implications for social work.'" *International Social Work*, 50 (5), 686–90.

Al-Krenawi, A. (1999). "Social workers practicing in their non-western home communities: Overcoming conflict between professional and cultural values." *Families in Society*, 80, 488–95.

British Association of Social Workers. (2001). "Code of ethics for social work." Retrieved from http://www.basw.co.uk/thankyou/coe/ (February 12, 2011)

Dubowitz, H. (2009). "Child protection around the world: Similarities and differences, advances and challenges." *International Journal of Child Health and Human Development*, 2, 217–22.

Fargion, S. (2008). "Reflections on social work's identity: International themes in Italian practitioners' representation of social work." *International Social Work*, 51, 206–19.

Gray, M., & Fook, J. (2004). "The quest for a universal social work: Some issues and implications." *Social Work Education*, 23, 625–44.

Hare, I. (2004). "Defining social work for the 21st century: The international federation of social workers' revised definition of social work." *International Social Work*, 47, 407–24.

Hendriks, P., Kloppenburg, R., Gevorgianiene, V., & Jakutiene, V. (2008). "Cross-national social work case analysis: Learning from international experience within an electronic environment." *European Journal of Social Work*, 11, 383–96.

International Federation of Social Workers (IFSW). (2000). "Definition of social work. General Meeting Montréal, Québec, Canada." Retrieved from http://www.ifsw.org/f38000138.html

Kniephoff-Knebel, A., & Seibel, F. (2008). "Establishing international cooperation in social work education: The first decade of the international committee of schools for social work (ICSSW)." *International Social Work*, 51, 780–12.

Kreitzer, L., & Wilson, M. (2010). "Shifting perspectives on international alliances in social work: Lessons from Ghana and Nicaragua." *International Social Work*, 53, 701–19.

Kohli, H. K., & Faul, A. C. (2005). "Cross-cultural differences towards diversity issues in attitudes of graduating social work students in India and the United States." *International Social Work*, 48, 809–22.

Lalayants, M., Tripodi, T., & Jung, S. (2009). "Trends in domestic and international social work research: A 10-year review of American research journals." *Journal of Social Service Research*, 35, 209–15.

Lindsey, E. W. (2005). "Study abroad and values development in social work students." *Journal of Social Work Education*, 41, 229–49.

Leung, J. B. (2007). "An international definition of social work for China." *International Journal of Social Welfare*, 16, 391–97.

Midgley, J. (2001). "Issues in international social work: Resolving critical debates in the profession." *Journal of Social Work*, 1, 21–35.

Miu Chung, Y. (2008). "Exploring cultural tensions in cross-cultural social work practice." *Social Work*, 53, 317–28.

Moldovan, V., & Moyo, O. (2007). "Contradictions in the ideologies of helping: Examples from Zimbabwe and Moldova." *International Social Work*, 50, 461–72.

National Association of Social Workers (NASW). (2008). "Preamble to the code of ethics." Retrieved February 12, 2011, from http://www.socialworkers.org/pubs/Code/code.asp

Parrott, L. (2009). Constructive marginality: COnflicts and dilemmas in cultural competence and anti-oppressive practice. *Social Work Education*, 28, 617–630.

Rasmusson, B., Hyvönen, U., Nygren, L., & Khoo, E. (2010). "Child-centered social work practice—three unique meanings in the context of looking after children and the assessment framework in Australia, Canada and Sweden." *Children & Youth Services Review*, 32, 452–59.

Saito, Y., & Johns, R. (2009). "Japanese students' perceptions of international perspectives in social work." *International Social Work*, 52, 60–71.

Stewart, C., & Koeske, G. (2006). "Social work students' attitudes concerning the use of religious and spiritual interventions in social work practice." *Journal of Teaching in Social Work*, 26, 31–49.

Toseland, R., & McClive-Reed, K. (2009). "Social group work: International and global perspectives." *Social Work with Groups*, 32, 5–13.

Weiss, I. (2006). "Modes of practice and the dual mission of social work: A cross-national study of social work students' preferences." *Journal of Social Service Research*, 32, 135–51.

Weiss-Gal, I., & Welbourne, P. (2008). "The professionalisation of social work: A cross-national exploration." *International Journal of Social Welfare*, 17, 281–90.

Index